SLIDE INTERPRETATION
IN
CLINICAL MEDICINE

SLIDE INTERPRETATION IN CLINICAL MEDICINE

Farrukh Iqbal
MBBS (Pb.), MD (USA)
MRCP (UK), FRCP (Edin), FRCP (London)
Professor of Medicine
Shaikh Zayed Postgraduate Medical Institute
Consultant Physician
Shaikh Zayed Hospital
Lahore 54600
Pakistan

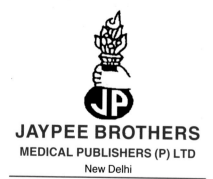

JAYPEE BROTHERS
MEDICAL PUBLISHERS (P) LTD
New Delhi

Published by

Jitendar P Vij

Jaypee Brothers Medical Publishers (P) Ltd

EMCA House, 23/23B Ansari Road, Daryaganj

New Delhi 110 002, India

Phones: +91-11-23272143, +91-11-23272703,
     +91-11-23282021, +91-11-23245672

Fax: +91-11-23276490, +91-11-23245683

e-mail: jaypee@jaypeebrothers.com

Visit our website: www.jaypeebrothers.com

Branches

- 202 Batavia Chambers, 8 Kumara Krupa Road
  Kumara Park East, **Bangalore** 560 001
  Phones: +91-80-22285971, +91-80-22382956, +91-80-30614073
  Tele Fax : +91-80-22281761   e-mail: jaypeebc@bgl.vsnl.net.in

- 282 IIIrd Floor, Khaleel Shirazi Estate, Fountain Plaza
  Pantheon Road, **Chennai** 600 008
  Phones: +91-44-28262665, +91-44-28269897 Fax: +91-44-28262331
  e-mail: jpmedpub@md3.vsnl.net.in

- 4-2-1067/1-3, 1st Floor, Balaji Building,
  Ramkote Cross Road, **Hyderabad** 500 095
  Phones: +91-40-55610020, +91-40-24758498 Fax: +91-40-24758499
  e-mail: jpmedpub@rediffmail.com

- 1A Indian Mirror Street, Wellington Square
  Kolkata 700 013, Phones: +91-33-22456075, +91-33-22451926
  Fax: +91-33-22456075   e-mail: jpbcal@cal.vsnl.net.in

- 106 Amit Industrial Estate, 61 Dr SS Rao Road
  Near MGM Hospital, Parel, **Mumbai** 400 012
  Phones: +91-22-24124863, +91-22-24104532, +91-22-30926896
  Fax: +91-22-24160828   e-mail: jpmedpub@bom7.vsnl.net.in

Slide Interpretation in Clinical Medicine

© 2006, Farrukh Iqbal

First Edition: **2006**

ISBN 81-8061-596-0

Typeset at JPBMP typesetting unit

Printed at Gopsons Papers Ltd, A-14, Sector 60, Noida 201 301, India

To
My wife Shahina,
my daughters,
Saliha and Zunaira and
my son, Aizad

FOREWORD

This book is not merely a slide show for "spot diagnosis".

It is a rich collection of slides of recognizable physical signs of disease, their complications and their relevant investigative procedures.

The slides range widely including almost all disciplines of internal medicine, from the commonest illnesses like measles, to those rarities like Thalidomide toxicity (unlikely to be seen again!). Hence it is a treasure trove, which has been compiled over many years with a great deal of care and industry.

What tremendously adds to the value of the book is the simulating questions with each slide, and is the only book of its type which describes the etiology, pathology, complications, differential diagnosis, treatment (even dosage and duration!) and prognosis of the "projected" disease where relevant.

The quality of the slides, the wealth of information and the selection of the material make it a "must" in the bookshelf of every postgraduate candidate and most physicians who will find enough material in it to refer to it again and again.

Prof Farrukh Iqbal, who is a prolific author, needs to be congratulated on this most commendable effort.

Khwaja Saadiq Husain
FRCP (Ed), FCPS (PAK), FCPS (BD), MAM (Malaysia)
Former
President
College of Physicians and Surgeons, Pakistan
Principal and Professor of Medicine
KE Medical College, Lahore
Dean, Faculty of Medicine
University of Punjab, Pakistan

PREFACE

Medicine is an ever changing field and every now and then new advances in the diagnosis and treatment of diseases take place. One should know the basic knowledge of the subject and to test that various techniques of examinations have developed over the past many years. These include essay writing, multiple choice questions, data interpretation, Objectively Structured Clinical Examination (OSCE) and recently introduced Task Oriented Assessment of Clinical Skills (TOACS) by the College of Physicians and Surgeons Pakistan for the FCPS-II Medicine examination.

This also includes showing some clinical slides to test the knowledge of the candidate. This book is an effort to assemble a few slides of clinically important diseases and investigations for the candidates to interpret and assess their knowledge to explain projected photographic material.

This book is designed as an aid for this examination and is the first of its kind in Pakistan. The format is very simple. There are 125 slides comprising clinical signs, X-rays and other radiological investigations. Each slide has few questions at the bottom and the answers are written overleaf. An effort has been made to make this book very simple and the author has tried to be precise as far as the answers are concerned. This book by no means can give all the current informations as regards the cases; however the candidate should consult the standard textbooks of medicine in the market.

One should sit back, relax with a cup of tea and go through this book swiftly, enjoy and at the same time assess their knowledge in medicine. It is advised that the reader should carefully read the main statement and then the questions and answer precisely. The author believes strongly that things once seen are hardly forgotten ever.

This book is the first of its series of four books on slides. I shall warmly welcome any valuable suggestions in improving the next issues.

In the end I wish good luck to the students for their examinations.

Farrukh Iqbal
E-mail: fiqbal56@hotmail.com

ACKNOWLEDGEMENTS

It gives me a great pleasure to acknowledge my colleagues and students for asking me to write this book and I think that without their continuous pursuance, it would have been a difficult task. I am thankful to Dr Asif Kamal, FRCP (Edin), FRCP (Lond), Consultant Physician in Lincoln County Hospital, Lincoln, UK for encouraging me to collect interesting slides and allowing me to follow his footsteps in academics. I am thankful to Dr Attya Mahboob, Associate Professor of Dermatology for reviewing questions pertaining to dermatology. I am also grateful to Mr Ajaz Ahmad (KPO) for typing the manuscript and for his helping attitude with always a smiling face.

CONTENTS

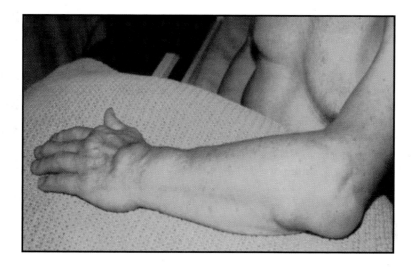

This patient had dryness of mouth and eyes.

1. What three abnormalities are present?
2. What is the primary diagnosis?
3. What four pulmonary complications can occur?

ANSWERS

1. The three abnormalities are:
   a. Swelling on the dorsum of left wrist (synovial thickening).
   b. Wasting of the small muscles of the hand (guttering).
   c. Nodular swelling at the elbow (nodules).
2. The primary diagnosis is rheumatoid arthritis.
3. The four pulmonary complications are as follows:
   a. Pleural effusion (exudative).
   b. Pulmonary fibrosis (fibrosing alveolitis).
   c. Rheumatoid nodules if patient is a miner, this complex is called Caplan's syndrome.
   d. Bronchiolitis obliterans.

Out of the above four, the first three will have restrictive pulmonary functions where as the last one has obstructive pulmonary function.

The reader should be careful in answering question 3, as there is a difference between pulmonary and intrathoracic complications. The later include cardiac and skeletal abnormalities.

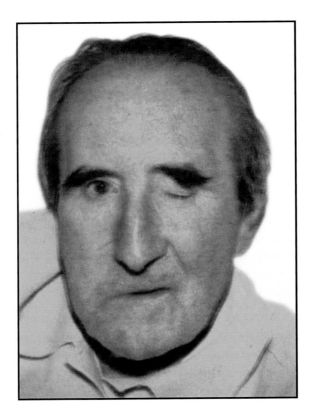

This 68-year-old man had right sided weakness.
1. What abnormalities are shown in this slide?
2. What is the diagnosis?
3. Name few other conditions in context to this problem.

ANSWERS

1. Following are the abnormalities:
   a. There is complete ptosis on the left (left oculomotor nerve palsy).
   b. There is prominent left nasolabial fold (right facial nerve palsy).
   c. There is already right-sided hemiplegia.
2. The diagnosis is Weber's syndrome, a type of crossed hemiplegia in which there is ipsilateral oculomotor nerve palsy (nuclear), contralateral facial nerve palsy (upper motor neuron type) and contralateral hemiplegia. The lesion is in the base of midbrain on the left side.
3. The other examples of crossed paralysis and similar brainstem lesions are as follows:
   a. *Claude's syndrome*: There is ipsilateral oculomotor palsy, with contralateral cerebellar ataxia and tremors. The lesion is in tegmentum of the midbrain.
   b. *Benedikt's syndrome*: There is ipsilateral oculomotor palsy, with contralateral cerebellar ataxia, tremors and corticospinal signs of midbrain. The lesion is in the tegmentum.
   c. *Parinaud's syndrome*: In this, supranuclear coordinating mechanism for upward gaze is involved along with fixed pupils and divergence of eyes. The lesion is in superior colliculus (tectum of the midbrain).
   d. *Millard-Gubler syndrome*: There is ipsilateral facial and abducens nerve palsy and contralateral hemiplegia. The lesion is in the base of pons.
   e. *Avellis syndrome*: There is ipsilateral vagal nerve palsy and contralateral hemiplegia. The lesion is in the tegmentum of medulla.
   f. *Jackson's syndrome*: There is ipsilateral vagus and hypoglossal nerve palsy and contralateral hemiplegia. The lesion is again in the tegmentum of medulla.
   g. *Wallenberg's syndrome Posterior Inferior Cerebellar Artery (PICA)*: There is ipsilateral involvement of trigeminal, glosso-pharyngeal, vagal and accessory nerves leading to palsy, ipsilateral Horner's syndrome and cerebellar ataxia with contralateral loss of pain and temperature sense. The lesion is in the tegmentum of medulla.

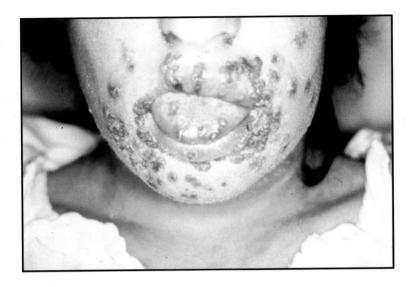

This young girl had fever.
1. Describe the abnormality in this slide.
2. What is the diagnosis?
3. What treatment could be offered?

ANSWERS

1. There are multiple, papulovesicular herpetiform lesions affecting the tongue, lips, perioral region and nose of this young girl.
2. The diagnosis is primary herpes simplex with superadded infection.
3. The treatment includes oral acyclovir 400 mg five times a day for 5-7 days or intravenously in a dose of 7.5-10 mg/kg in three divided doses daily for 5-7 days.

Amoxicillin and clavulanic acid (Augmentin) can be given orally to treat superadded infection.

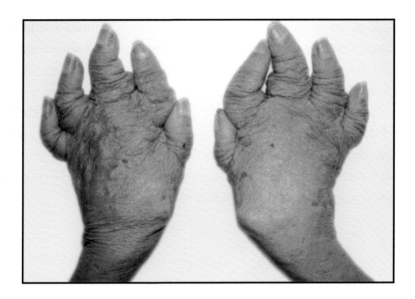

This patient had an itchy rash over her elbows and knees.
1. Describe the abnormality.
2. What name is given to this deformity?
3. What is the underlying diagnosis?
4. What is telescoping sign?

ANSWERS

1. There is gross deformity of both hands with ulnar deviation, (resembling rheumatoid arthritis), distortion and shortening of digits (underlying osteolysis).
2. Arthritis mutilans.
3. Psoriatic arthritis as the itchy rash over elbows and knees (extensor surfaces) is due to psoriasis.
4. If the digit is stretched from the distal end there is lengthening which on releasing goes back to its previous position. This is called telescoping sign as in old-fashioned telescopes.

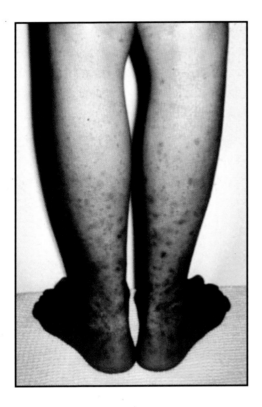

This young boy had pain in abdomen and developed a rash as shown in the slide.

1. Describe the rash.
2. What do you expect to see in the urine?
3. Why this boy has abdominal pain?
4. What is the underlying diagnosis?

ANSWERS

1. Multiple, erythematous lesions of few millimeters to a centimeter in size are present on calves and dorsum of feet.
2. Microscopic or macroscopic haematuria and proteinuria.
3. The abdominal pain is due to vasculitis of intestinal tract, (associated with bleeding). Intussusception of intestine also causes acute pain and is palpable as a sausage shaped swelling.
4. The diagnosis is Henoch-Schönlein purpura affecting the skin and intestinal tract.

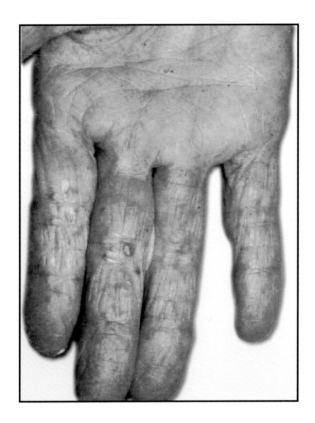

This patient was a smoker and asymptomatic.

1. Describe the abnormality.
2. What name is given to this abnormality?
3. What is its significance?

ANSWERS

1. There are multiple, bluish, tortuous veins on the palmar aspect of fingers and adjacent portion of palm while pulps of digits are red and are spared.
2. Venous varicosities.
3. Mostly insignificant.

   NB: It is sometimes difficult to differentiate from cyanosis but the pulps of the fingers are not cyanosed.

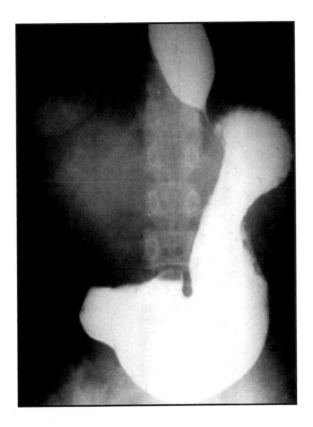

This patient had difficulty in swallowing.
1. What is this investigation?
2. What abnormality is shown?
3. What is the diagnosis?
4. What is the treatment?

ANSWERS

1. This is a barium meal.
2. There is dilatation of oesophagus, absent peristalsis, poor oesophageal emptying and smooth symmetrical tapering of the distal oesophagus like a "rat tail" or "bird's beak".
3. Achalasia of the cardia.
4. The treatment is:
   a. Endoscopically guided injection of botulinum toxin (relapse is common).
   b. Pneumatic dilatation with balloon (perforation rate < 3%).
   c. Surgical myotomy (modified Heller's cardiomyotomy) has excellent results (>85%) but gastro-oesophageal reflux is common. Fundoplication along with this procedure can help reflux.

SLIDE - 8

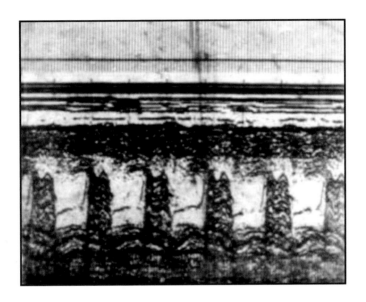

This patient had sudden loss of vision in his right eye.
1. What is this investigation?
2. What does it show?
3. What is the diagnosis?
4. What is the treatment?

ANSWERS

1. This is a B-mode echocardiogram.
2. It shows normal E-F slope, wide space between anterior and posterior mitral valve leaflets and homogeneous multiple echoes between these leaflets. (Vegetations due to infective endocarditis are shown as heterogeneous echoes).
3. Left atrial myxoma.
4. The treatment is surgical excision of the myxoma. It is usually curative.

NB: Occasionally, transthoracic echocardiography may miss tumours; therefore MRI will be a better option. On auscultation, there is a tumour plop due to a diastolic sound related to tumour movement.

Patients with myxoma can present with a picture mimicking a systemic illness and signs of peripheral embolization.

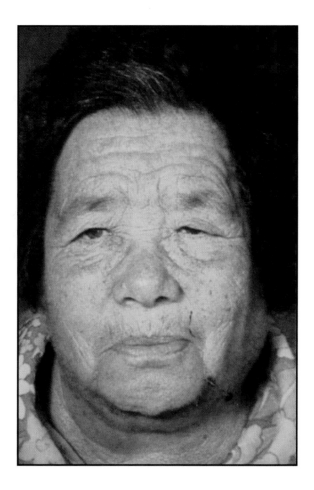

This patient was hard of hearing and had been found to be hypothermic.

1. Describe the abnormalities on this slide.
2. How this patient would present to a cardiologist, neurologist and gastroenterologist?
3. What is the diagnosis?
4. What is the treatment?

ANSWERS

1. The abnormalities are:
   a. Puffiness of the face.
   b. Pale complexion.
   c. Coarsening of hair and facial features.
   d. Scanty eyebrows.
2. This patient can present to:
   a. Cardiologist for dyspnoea or chest pain.
   b. Neurologist for weakness, myalgias, muscle cramps, numbness, dysarthria, headache, decreased sense of taste and smell and gait disorder.
   c. Gastroenterologist for anorexia and severe constipation.
3. Hypothyroidism.
4. The treatment is replacement with thyroxine. In a young patient one can start with a little bit higher dose, i.e. 50 to 100 µg daily for a couple of weeks then increased by 25 ug every 1-3 weeks until the patient is euthyroid.

   In an old patient with underlying coronary heart disease, the dose should be 25 ug daily for two weeks then increased by 25 ug at 1-3 week's interval until the patient is euthyroid.

   Repeat thyroid function tests are mandatory. Most of these patients are maintained on 100-250 µg of thyroxine daily.

   NB: If a hypothyroid patient does not respond to conventional thyroxine treatment, then concomitant adrenal insufficiency should be ruled out.

SLIDE - 10

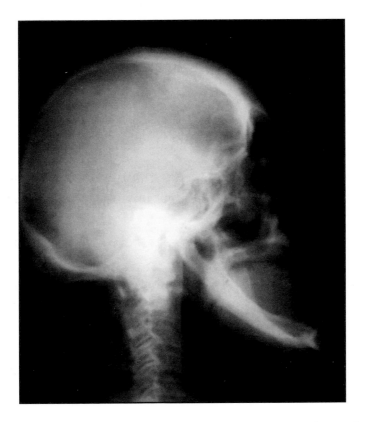

This patient complained of headaches, sweating and was found to have hypertension.

1. What is shown in this slide?
2. What is the diagnosis?
3. Name two laboratory and one clinical test to confirm the diagnosis.

ANSWERS

1. This is a slide of X-ray skull, lateral view. It shows enlarged skull, prominent frontal sinuses (frontal bossing), wide pituitary fossa, and protruding lower jaw (prognathism).
2. Acromegaly.
3. The laboratory tests are:
   a. Elevated growth hormone / elevated insulin like growth factor-1 (IGF-1).
   b. Non-suppression of serum growth hormone by oral glucose. The clinical test is perimetry to find any visual field defects.

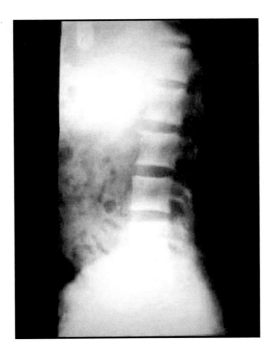

This X-ray belongs to a patient who is known to have chronic renal failure.

1. What abnormality is shown in this picture?
2. What name is given to this abnormality?
3. How do you prevent this?

ANSWERS

1. There is decreased bone density in the middle of each vertebra and this along with intervertebral spaces appears as alternate white and dark bands.
2. Rugger Jersy spine – named after the uniform kit for rugby players.
3. This is due to renal osteodystrophy, which results due to chronic renal failure. There is decreased hydroxylation of vitamin D to 1,25 dihydroxy cholecalciferol (activated vitamin D) leading to hypocalcaemia and secondary hyperparathyroidism. Therefore, treatment of renal failure, and supplementation of vitamin D (activated form) and calcium are the mainstay of the management. Reduction of phosphates by giving calcium acetate may also help.

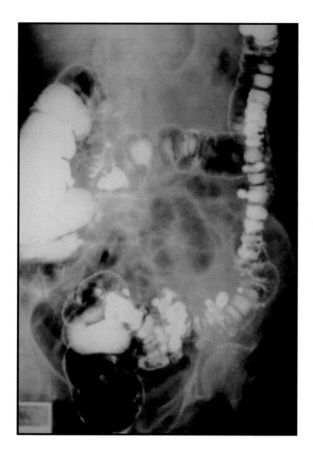

This patient had bleeding per rectum.
1. What is this investigation?
2. What does it show?
3. What is the diagnosis?
4. What is the management?

ANSWERS

1. This is a double contrast barium enema.
2. It shows multiple out pocketing containing contrast in the descending and sigmoid colon.
3. Diverticulosis.
4. Half of the cases of acute lower gastrointestinal bleeding are attributable to diverticulosis. Although diverticulae are more on the left side but bleeding occurs more common from the right side. It presents as acute, painless, large volume maroonish or bright red hematochezia in patients age over 50. Important considerations include the following:
   a. Exclude upper GI bleeding by passing a nasogastric tube.
   b. Anoscopy (or proctoscopy) and sigmoidoscopy should be performed.
   c. Colonoscopy is performed to determine the site of bleeding and it should be performed within 6-24 hours.
   d. Small intestine push enteroscopy or capsule imaging (video pill) is a newly emerging technology.
   e. Nuclear bleeding scans and angiography to localize site of bleeding.

Following steps are taken:
a. Discontinue aspirin or non-steroidal anti-inflammatory drugs (NSAIDs) if the patient is already taking.
b. Check complete blood count and clotting profile.
c. Arrange blood transfusion at least 4 units of blood.
d. Therapeutic sigmoidoscopy/colonoscopy for epinephrine injection, cautery or metallic clips or laser.
e. Intra-arterial vasopressin or embolization can be done selectively. Intra-arterial embolization is preferred.
f. Surgical intervention is needed if all of the above modalities fail. However, before surgical procedure, localization of bleeding point is mandatory. Different types of hemicolectomies with suitable anastomoses are recommended.

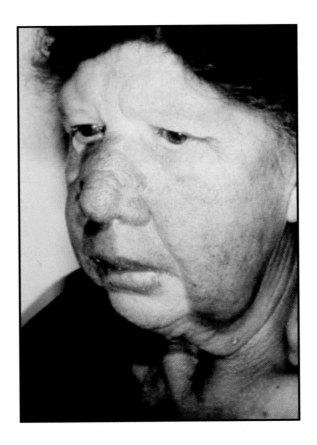

This patient had renal stones and arthralgia.

1. Describe the abnormality on this slide.
2. What name is given to this abnormality?
3. What is the diagnosis?

ANSWERS

1. Skin over the nose, cheeks, upper lip and supraorbital region of this lady is thick and of dusky red to violaceous in colour.
2. She may be a case of sarcoidosis. Involvement of tip of the nose is called lupus pernio.
3. Histopathological examination of the skin is required.

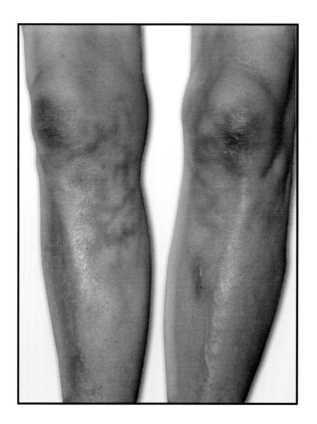

This patient was hypothyroid.

1. Describe the abnormality in this slide.
2. What name is given to this abnormality?
3. How does it differ from another skin rash which occurs in autoimmune disorders?

ANSWERS

1. Brown-red macular lesions in reticulate pattern are present on both the shins.
2. Erythema ab igne.
3. The similar skin rash is livedo reticularis which occurs in auto-immune disorders, e.g. polyarteritis nodosa.

Erythema ab igne is dark brown, with lacy pattern and occurs due to denaturation of haemoglobin in the subcutaneous vessels due to heat as these patients sit in front of fire due to feeling of excessive cold. This cannot be blanched with pressure either, as these are permanent. Ulceration may be present due to heat and skin damage especially if there is also an element of neuropathy (e.g. diabetics). However, livedo reticularis is most apparent on thighs and in warm weather it disappears. It is of fish net pattern with reticulated cyanotic areas surrounding pale central core. It can be blanched with pressure. Usually, there is no ulceration.

SLIDE - 15

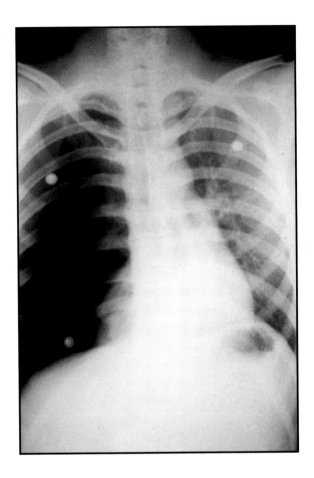

This man was brought to accident and emergency department with a history of severe sudden chest pain while playing football.

1. What are the abnormalities in this slide?
2. What is the diagnosis?
3. How would you manage this patient?

ANSWERS

1. The abnormalities on this slide are:
   a. There is hyperlucent right hemithorax.
   b. There are no visible lung markings.
   c. The mediastinum is shifted to left side.
   d. Electrodes for monitoring are visible.
   e. The right hemi-diaphragm is lower than the left hemi-diaphragm.
2. Right sided tension pneumothorax.
3. As it is tension pneumothorax, therefore, insertion of a wide bore needle in the right hemithorax through any (preferably in the right second intercostal space) intercostal space should be the first step. One could hear a gush of air or a whistling sound due to release of trapped air under tension and patient feels relaxed after the trapped air is let out. After this, the patient should under go chest tube placement (tube thoracostomy). If the expansion is complete, then follow-up is necessary, otherwise surgical intervention is required.

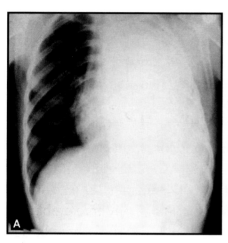 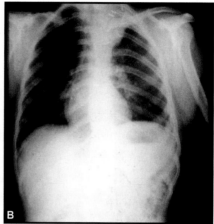

These chest X-rays are from a 12-year-old boy who presented with severe dyspnoea, was anaemic and had bilateral axillary freckling.

1. What is shown in A?
2. What is shown in B?
3. What is the primary diagnosis?
4. What complication had occurred?

ANSWERS

1. There is complete homogenous opacification of left hemithorax probably due to massive pleural effusion.
2. There is rounded homogenous opacity in the left upper zone adjacent to the superior mediastinum. A few opaque elongated shadows are also seen in that opacity.
3. Neurofibrosarcoma.
4. This patient had axillary freckling and left sided pleural effusion, which was drained and was uniformly blood stained. The patient had neurofibromatosis, and one of the paraspinal neurofibroma had transformed into neurofibrosarcoma. The dense elongated opacities are yttrium needles for brachy-radiotherapy for neurofibrosarcoma. Axillary freckling is pathognomonic sign of neurofibromatosis or von Recklinghausen's disease.

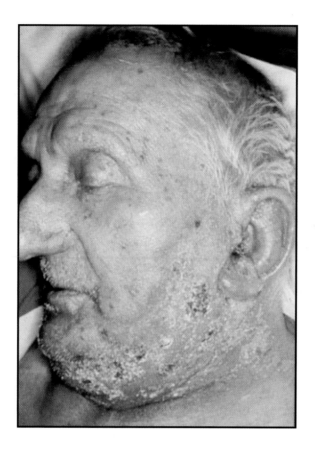

This patient had chronic lymphocytic leukaemia (CLL) and had a painful rash on his face as shown in the slide.

1. What is the abnormality?
2. What is the diagnosis?
3. What is the treatment?
4. Name one most important complication.

ANSWERS

1. Ulcerated, crusted lesions are present on the left lower face and left ear in the distribution of mandibular branch of the left trigeminal nerve.
2. Herpes zoster of mandibular division of left trigeminal nerve.
3. General measures include isolation of the patient until primary crusts have disappeared. Skin needs to keep clean, antihistamines for pruritus and analgesics for pain are recommended. Topical antiviral cream or antibiotic ointments can be applied.

   Specific measures include antiviral therapy with acyclovir 7.5-10 mg/kg IV for 2-3 days then orally 800 mg 5 times a day for 5 days or valacyclovir 1000 mg thrice a day or famciclovir 500 mg thrice a day for 7-10 days. Role of corticosteroids is controversial. Secondary bacterial infection is treated with antibiotics. This patient has underlying immunocompromised status due to chronic lymphocytic leukaemia.
4. The most important complication is post-herpetic neuralgia which can be treated with:
   a. Non-steroidal anti-inflammatory drugs (NSAID's).
   b. Tricyclic antidepressants.
   c. Lidocaine patches (local slow release anaesthetic).
   d. Carbamazepine can be given up to 1200 mg per day in divided doses.
   e. Gabapentin from 300 mg daily to 3600 mg daily in divided doses.
   f. Alcohol injection in the nerves for neuronal block.
   g. Dorsal rhizotomy.
   h. Accupuncture.

SLIDE - 18

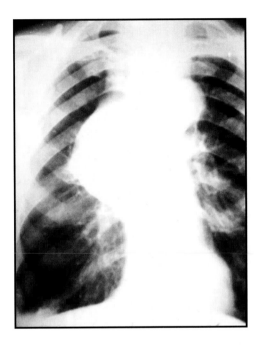

This patient presented with chest pain not responding to usual anti-anginal therapy.

    1. What abnormality is shown in this slide?

    2. What is the most likely diagnosis?

    3. What is the treatment?

ANSWERS

1. There is bulging on the right side of the superior mediastinum which seems originating from the ascending aorta.
2. The most likely diagnosis with the history of chest pain not responding to conventional antianginal therapy is dissection of ascending aorta/aortic aneurysm.
3. The hypertension should be controlled by rapidly acting anti-hypertensive agent, i.e. nitroprusside (50 mg in 1000 ml of 5% dextrose in water, at a rate of 0.5 ml/min which is increased by 0.5 ml every 5 minutes. Serum thiocyanate levels should be obtained, if treatment is to continue for 48 hours. The infusion is stopped if the drug level reaches 10 mg/dl. The other agent used is intravenous propranolol 0.15 mg/ kg over 5 minutes and repeated if necessary. If dissection is distal to aortic valve, it is called type A, and if distal to left subclavian artery it is called type B. For type A, aortic valve and arch are replaced with re-attachment of the coronaries and brachiocephalic vessels. Mortality is 20% after the operation. For type B, the operation may be delayed until the BP is controlled and dissection has been established. Surgery is then planned. Mortality is higher than type A. All un-operated patients should be followed with annual CT scan to detect progressive enlargement.

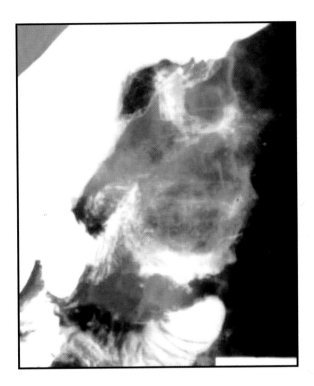

This picture is from a 60 years old lady who presented with anaemia, low grade fever and an epigastric mass.

1. What is this investigation?
2. What does it show?
3. Why is this patient anaemic?

ANSWERS

1. This is a barium meal examination radiograph.
2. It shows normal contour of lesser curvature but at greater curvature there is a huge filling defect with barium scattered in pockets. Part of the swelling is also protruding in to the cavity of stomach with a crater.
3. The anaemia is due to chronic blood loss in the intestinal tract. This swelling was biopsied and was found to be a leiomyosarcoma of the stomach, which is a rare entity. However, leiomyomas are more common and one of them can transform into sarcoma.

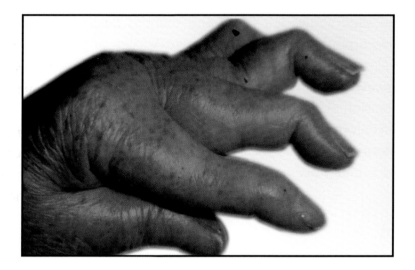

This patient complained of morning stiffness of her fingers.
1. Describe the abnormality shown in this slide.
2. What name is given to this?
3. What is the primary diagnosis?

ANSWERS

1. The slide shows left hand and there is flexion of digits at metacarpophalangeal joints, hyperextension at proximal inter-phalangeal joints and flexion at distal interphalangeal joints. However, there is flexion of 1st metacarpophalangeal joint and extension at interphalangeal joint of the thumb.
2. The deformity of digits is called "swan neck deformity" while the deformity of thumb is called "Z-deformity".
3. The primary diagnosis is rheumatoid arthritis.

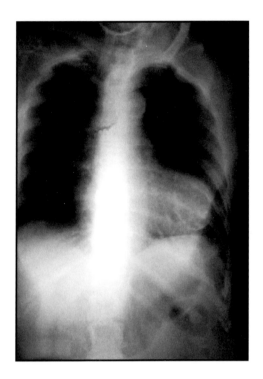

This patient had breathlessness on exertion and a week ago had right hemiplegia.

1. Describe the abnormality shown in this slide.
2. What is the diagnosis?
3. What would you see in the ECG?

ANSWERS

1. This chest radiograph shows enlargement of the left ventricle almost extending to the lateral chest wall. The tip of the ventricle shows opacity with a calcified ring.
2. Left ventricular aneurysm with a calcified thrombus
3. The ECG shows persistent elevation of the ST segment with convexity upwards and deep Q-waves indicating previous infarction in the lateral chest leads.

SLIDE - 22

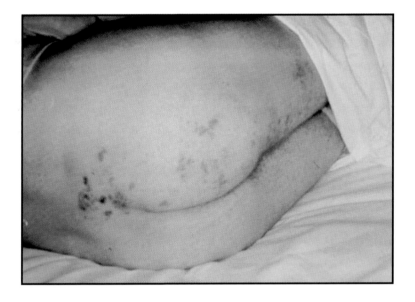

This patient is a diabetic and developed a painful rash.
1. What is this rash?
2. What complications this patient can develop?
3. What is the treatment?

ANSWERS

1. There are clusters of crusted vesicles distributed unilaterally in the distribution of sacral dermatomes, S_2, S_3 and S_4. This rash is due to herpes zoster.
2. Sacral herpes zoster can lead to bowel and bladder dysfunction. Incidence of post-herpetic neuralgia is high in diabetics.
3. The treatment includes early antiviral therapy, i.e. acyclovir 800 mg five times daily. Famciclovir 500 mg thrice daily, valacyclovir 1000 mg thrice daily. All these agents are given for 7-10 days
   - Antibiotics are added to prevent super added bacterial infections.
   - Non-steroidal anti-inflammatory drugs (NSAID's) are used to relieve pain.
   - Antiviral or antibiotic preparations can be applied topically.

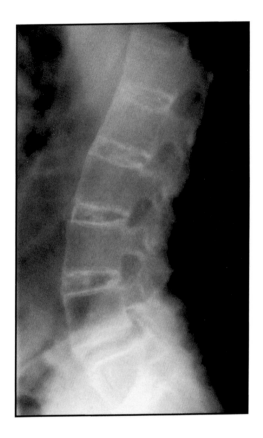

This 45-year-old man had low back pain for the last few years.
1. Describe the abnormality.
2. What name is given to this abnormality?
3. What is the diagnosis?
4. Mention four remote complications.

ANSWERS

1. There is involvement of apophyseal joints of the spine, ossification of annulus fibrosis, calcification of the anterior and posterior spinal ligaments, squaring of vertebrae and generalized demineralization of the vertebral bodies.
2. The name "bamboo spine" has been used to describe the late radiographic appearance of the spinal column.
3. The diagnosis is ankylosing spondylitis.
4. The remote complications include:
   a. Spondylitic heart disease characterised by conduction defects and aortic insufficiency (3-5%).
   b. Non-granulomatous anterior uveitis (25%).
   c. Pulmonary fibrosis, cavitation and bronchiectasis.
   d. Transient acute arthritis of peripheral joints (50%).
   Ankylosing spondylitis and ulcerative colitis have close association.

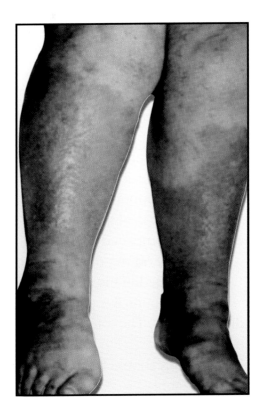

This patient was losing weight in spite of a good appetite. She also complained of excessive sweating and frequent loose stools.

1. What is the abnormality?
2. What is the diagnosis?
3. Name two other components of the disease.
4. What is the treatment?

ANSWERS

1. There is thickening of the skin over the shins.
2. Pre-tibial myxoedema.
3. This patient has Grave's disease as she is losing weight inspite of a good appetite and also has excessive sweating. The triad consists of pretibial myxoedema, exophthalmos and diffuse goitre.
4. The treatment includes:
    a. Propranolol for symptomatic relief. Dose as high as 80 mg four times a day can be used.
    b. Carbimazole or propyl thiouracil are good for old patients but there is high rate of relapse of thyrotoxicosis. At least 2 years of therapy should be completed.

Carbimazole is used as 30-60 mg once a day or spaced out in three doses. It is usually stopped in the last month of pregnancy to avoid foetal goitre. Propyl thiouracil is given in a dose of 300-600 mg daily in four divided doses. The total dose during pregnancy is kept below 200 mg per day.

Side effects of these drugs should be remembered.

- Iodinated contrast agents.
- Radioactive Iodine (^{131}I). It should not be given to pregnant women. Otherwise it is considered treatment of choice if there are no contraindications. It is less expensive, simple to administer and without side effects. However, sometimes the patients have to be given thyroxine supplements to avoid hypothyroidism.
- Thyroid surgery is usually preferred for pregnant women or those patients who are non-compliant to medicines or who have side effects from anti-thyroid drugs. Other indications include large goitres or if there is a significant chance of malignancy. Patients should be rendered euthyroid by a thiourea, ipodate sodium or lugol's iodine. Preoperatively, propranolol can be given to avoid thyroid crisis.

Complications of thyroid surgery should be avoided i.e. recurrent laryngeal nerve damage, hypoparathyroidism, etc.

SLIDE - 25

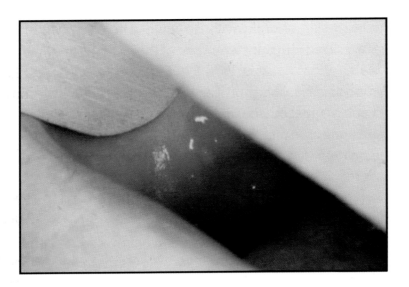

This slide is from a 5-year-old boy with a history of high grade fever and a skin rash.

1. What is shown in this slide?
2. What name is given to this abnormality?
3. What is the diagnosis?
4. How would you treat?

ANSWERS

1. The inner side of oral cavity is shown. There is a whitish area over a dull red mucous membrane of the cheek as tiny "table salt crystals".
2. This is called Koplik's spot. The other sites are lower conjunctival fold and vaginal mucous membrane.
3. The diagnosis is measles.
4. The treatment includes general measures, e.g. isolation for one week following onset of rash and bed rest until afebrile.

Other modalities include vitamin A 400,000 IU orally per day to maintain epithelial mucosa and immune enhancement. Secondary infections are treated with antibiotics and antipyretics. Post-measles encephalitis including Subacute Sclerosing Panencephalitis (SSPE) can only be treated symptomatically.

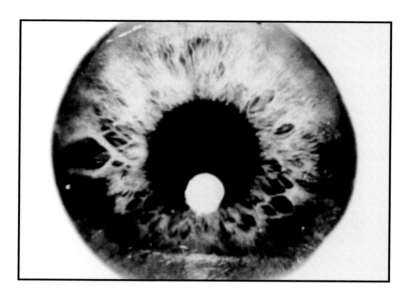

This patient had mental retardation and involuntary movements of his limbs. On examination, he was mildly jaundiced.

1. What abnormality is shown in this slide?
2. What is the primary diagnosis?
3. What is the mode of inheritance?
4. What three investigations would you ask for?
5. What is the treatment?

ANSWERS

1. There is brownish ring involving the periphery of cornea due to fine pigmented granular deposits in the Descemet's membrane close to endothelial surface. This is called Kayser-Fleischer ring.
2. Wilson's disease or hepatolenticular degeneration.
3. It is autosomal recessive disorder. The genetic defect is localized to chromosome 13 which involves a copper transporting enzyme, adenosine triphosphate (ATP 7B) in the liver.
4. The laboratory findings include the following:
   • Increased urinary copper excretion (> 100 mg/24h).
   • Low serum ceruloplasmin < 20 mg/ dl).
   • Elevated hepatic copper concentration (> 250 mg/ g of dry liver).
5. The treatment should start only before it causes neurologic or hepatic damage. This includes:
   • Restriction of copper containing foods, i.e. shellfish, organic food and legumes.
   • Penicillamine (0.75 – 2g/d) in divided doses.
   • Pyridoxine, 50 mg per week.
   • Trientine (if penicillamine is not tolerated) 250-500 mg thrice daily.
   • Oral zinc acetate 50 mg thrice daily promotes faecal copper excretion.
   • Ammonium tetra thiomolybdate has been useful as initial therapy for neurologic Wilson's disease.

   Treatment is continued indefinitely.

   Liver transplantation considered for fulminant hepatitis, end stage cirrhosis or intractable neurologic disease.

   Family members should be screened with ceruloplasmin levels, liver function tests and slit-lamp examinations.

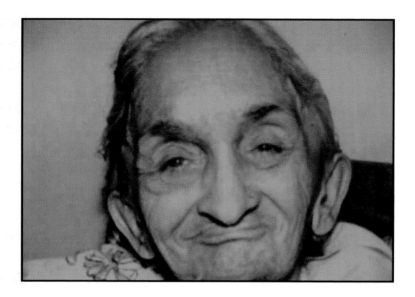

This 75-year-old lady was hard of hearing and complained pain in her left thigh.

1. What abnormality is shown in this slide?
2. What is the diagnosis?
3. Name seven complications of this disease.
4. Name few peripheral markers of this disease.

ANSWERS

1. There is protrusion of the vault of skull at the left temporal area with prominent vessels. There are also dilated superficial temporal vessels on the right temporal area. The skull seems asymmetrical and enlarged.
2. The diagnosis is Paget's disease of bone in view of the appearance and the fact that this patient is deaf and has pain in her left thigh, which may be due to involvement of left femur or fissure fracture.
3. The seven complications are:
   i. Bone pain.
   ii. Pathological fracture or fissure fractures.
   iii. Vertebral collapse leading to kyphosis or scoliosis and spinal cord compression.
   iv. Hyperdynamic heart failure.
   v. Entrapment neuropathies especially the nerves passing through ostial foramina, i.e. vestibular nerve, optic nerve or even spinal cord at foramen magnum in platybasia.
   vi. Development of osteogenic sarcoma if the disease is of more than 10 years duration. The overall incidence is 1%.
   vii. Hypercalcaemia leading to renal stone formation.
4. These include:
   • Raised serum alkaline phosphatase.
   • Elevated urinary hydroxyproline excretion.

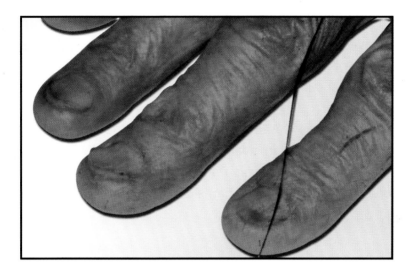

This patient had difficulty in swallowing and was also breathless on exertion.

1. What abnormality is shown?
2. How would you confirm it?
3. What is the diagnosis?
4. Why this patient has dysphagia?

ANSWERS

1. The nails of these digits are flattened and have become even concave, i.e. like a spoon called koilonychia.
2. If a drop of water is placed over these nails, it will not spill whereas in normally curved nails the drop cannot stabilize over the nail plate.
3. The diagnosis is Plummer-Winson's syndrome as this patient has anaemia, difficulty in swallowing and is breathless on exertion.
4. The dysphagia is due to the presence of oesophageal webs. However, a minority of patients develop post-cricoid carcinoma and can result in dysphagia.

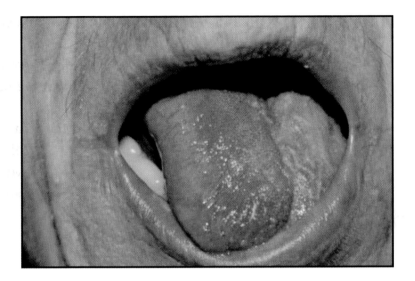

This 65-year-old patient had weight loss and is trying to protrude his tongue.

1. What two abnormalities do you see in this slide?
2. What is wrong with him?
3. Where is the lesion?

ANSWERS

1. The two abnormalities are:
   a. The tongue is deviated to the left side.
   b. The left half of the tongue is looking pale, less bulky and has folds or rugae similar to the appearance of "scrotal tongue".
2. There is left sided hypoglossal nerve palsy.
3. The lesion is in the path of the left hypoglossal nerve (nuclear or infra nuclear).

NB: In this case, the patient underwent removal of stone from the left submandibular gland but unfortunately the left hypoglossal nerve was damaged as it has a close relation with submandibular gland.

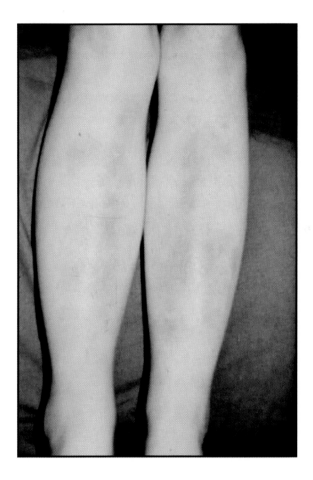

This young female had sore throat and developed these lesions.
1. Describe the lesions.
2. What name is given to it?
3. Name few causes of this abnormality.

ANSWERS

1. There are multiple round to oval, red nodules of variable size on the front of both shins. They are not ulcerated. The rest of shins are normal looking.
2. Erythema nodosum. These lesions regress slowly over several weeks to resemble contusions or bruises.
3. The causes include:
   - Infections, e.g. streptococcal, coccidioidomycosis, tuberculosis, Yersinia enterocolitica, syphilis and leprosy.
   - Inflammatory bowel diseases, e.g. ulcerative colitis, Crohn's disease.
   - Sarcoidosis.
   - Pregnancy and use of contraceptive pills.
   - Sulphonamides and other drugs.

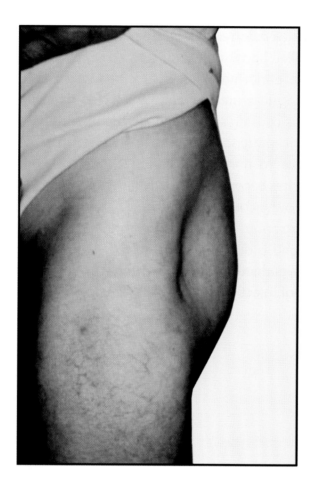

This is a 35-year-old diabetic who is on some treatment.
1. What abnormality is shown?
2. What name is given to this abnormality?
3. What may be the complications?

ANSWERS

1. There is excavation and depressed area on the left gluteal region.
2. This is called lipoatrophy.
3. There are abnormal vessels subcutaneously and if insulin is injected in these areas, it can be injected directly into a blood vessel thus causing severe hypoglycaemia. Insulin injection can cause both lipohypotrophy and lipohypertropy. The lipoatrophy occurs due to immune reaction to beef or pork insulin but incidence has become less due to the use of more purified insulins. Injection of this pure insulin directly in these areas can result in lipohypertrophy and restoration of normal contours. Lipo-hypertrophy is due to pharmacological effect of insulin. It can occur with purified insulins as well and the treatment is liposuction. Rotation of injection sites will prevent lipohypertrophy.

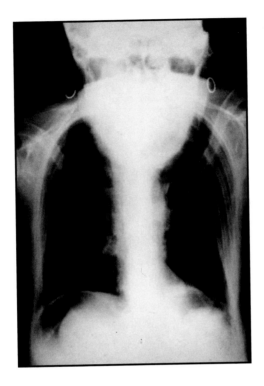

This 73-year-old lady presented to accident and emergency department with severe abdominal pain and vomiting.

1. Describe the abnormality.
2. What might have happened?
3. What is the treatment?

ANSWERS

1. This is a chest X-ray PA view showing air under the right dome of diaphragm. The opaque shadow above the clavicles is the stooped head of the patient.
2. She might have perforated a hollow viscus, i.e. gastric or duodenal ulcer, gallbladder, small bowel or large bowel, i.e. a diverticulum or a stercoral ulcer.
3. These include general measures including admission of the patient, intravenous fluids, nasogastric tube insertion and use of antibiotics. The antibiotic of choice is a third generation cephalosporin, e.g. cefotaxime (2 gm IV 8-12 hourly depending on renal functions). Ampicillin may be added if enterococcus is suspected. Metronidazole 500 mg IV 8 hourly can also be added.

Perforation of stomach can occur on the anterior wall of duodenum. If hypotension is present early, one should also consider the possibility of rupture of a major blood vessel.

The surgical treatment depends on rate of deterioration of the condition. Urgent laparotomy and closure of perforation with an omental patch called Graham's procedure with selective vagotomy may be a better option.

Nowadays laparoscopic closure of perforation can be performed in many centres reducing morbidity and mortality.

Up to 40% of such ulcers seal spontaneously. In poor operative candidates conservative management is required. Patient should be monitored closely while receiving fluids, continuous nasogastric suction, anti-secretory agents and broad-spectrum antibiotics.

If the condition deteriorates, surgery should be performed without delay.

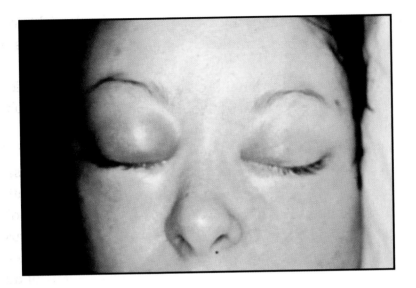

This patient was diabetic and presented with high grade fever, vomiting and headaches.

1. What is the abnormality?
2. What is the diagnosis?
3. What is the treatment?

ANSWERS

1. There is swelling, reddening of the right eyelid with proptosis. The right cheek is also swollen. The left eye is also swollen and is red on the inner side.
2. Right cavernous sinus thrombosis with probable extension to the left. The other associations are ophthalmoplegia, chemosis and visual loss. There may also be evidence of third, fourth, ophthalmic division of fifth and sixth cranial nerves. It should be differentiated from mucormycosis, which causes similar clinical picture.
3. The treatment is urgent and includes:
    a. Use of antibiotic against coagulase positive staphylococci and gram-negative pathogens.
    b. Anticoagulants have been used but their role is debatable.
    Antibiotics include flucloxacillin, amoxicillin+clavulanic acid, cephalosporins, e.g. cephazolin, vancomycin and methicillin, etc.

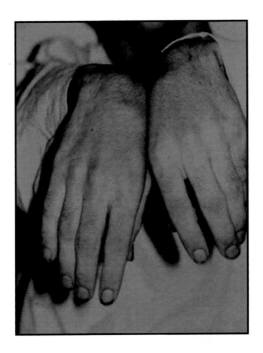

This patient was a painter by profession and is trying to dorsiflex his both hands.

1. What abnormality is shown in this slide?
2. What name is given to that?
3. What other complications he can develop?

ANSWERS

1. This slide shows that both hands are drooped forward. There is also minimal wasting of muscles of the dorsum of hands.
2. This is called bilateral wrist drop and is due to lead poisoning leading to motor neuropathy as this patient is a painter by profession and paint contains lead.
3. Other complications include colicky abdominal pain, constipation, headache, irritability, coma and convulsions. Chronic intoxication can cause learning disorders in children and of course motor neuropathy.

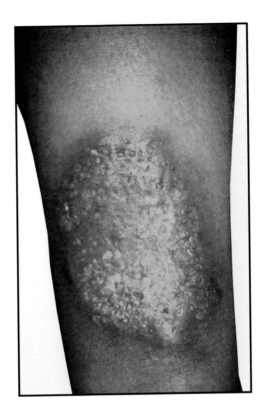

This patient had frequent bloody diarrhoea.

1. What is shown here?
2. What is the primary diagnosis?
3. What is the prognosis?

ANSWERS

1. This slide shows a large oval necrotic lesion in front of the shin. The lesion is indurated with multiple small openings with underlying micro abscesses. There is abundant necrotic material with pus formation. The rim is raised and is purplish in colour.
2. This is pyoderma gangrenosum and the underlying primary diagnosis is inflammatory bowel disease, probably ulcerative colitis.
3. Rapidly progressive lesions require systemic steroids, i.e. prednisolone 80-100 mg in divided doses. Some times azathioprine may be used in combination with steroids or alone.

   Tetracycline, colchicine and clofazimine have been shown to be of benefit in some patients. Topical and intralesional steroids may also help in indolent ulcers.

   Treatment of underlying cause usually results in spontaneous resolution of the lesion.

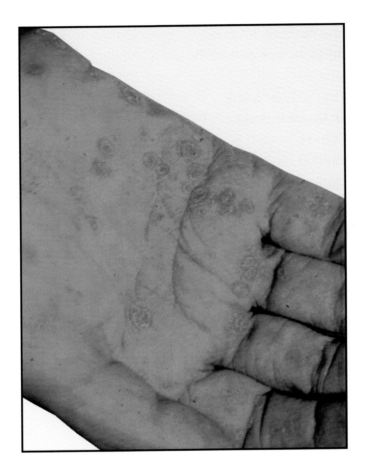

This patient was symptomatic.
1. Describe the lesions.
2. What are they?
3. What is the treatment?

ANSWERS

1. There are multiple, rounded 2-3 mm diameter well-circumscribed hyperkeratotic lesions over the palm and the fingers with a central dark area.
2. These are palmar warts.
3. The treatment includes:
   a. Cryotherapy with liquid nitrogen.
   b. Keratolytic agents, i.e. salicylic acid.
   c. Podophyllin resin.
   d. Imiquimod—5% cream of local interferon.
   e. Laser therapy—CO_2 laser is used.
   f. Retinoids.
   g. Bleomycin topically.

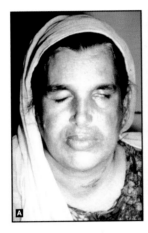 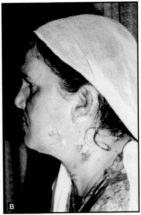 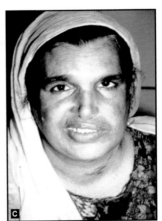

These three slides are from the same patient who developed hyperacusis in her left ear after a rash over the pinna of the left ear.

1. What is shown in slides A, B and C?
2. What is the diagnosis?
3. Why is she complaining of hyperacusis?

ANSWERS

1. Slide A shows left Bell's phenomenon (eyeball rolls up when the patient is asked to close the eye).

   Slide B shows a vesicular, ulcerated rash over the left side of the neck and left lower jaw. The left pinna also shows swelling and vesicular lesions.

   Slide C shows that the left nasolabial fold is less prominent than the right and mouth is deviated to the right side.

2. The diagnosis is left Ramsay Hunt syndrome, which is due to herpes zoster of the left geniculate ganglion.

3. The stapedius muscle is supplied by facial nerve when it passes through the middle ear. Once paralyzed, stapes is not pulled out and continuous vibrations leads to hyperacusis.

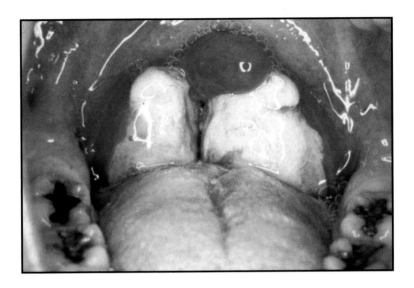

This young girl presented with fever, sore throat and difficulty in swallowing.

1. Describe the abnormalities.
2. What is the diagnosis?
3. How would you differentiate from a deadly infectious disease?
4. What is the treatment?

ANSWERS

1. The inside of oral cavity is shown in this slide. It shows that the uvula is swollen, the peritonsillar pillars are congested and tonsils are enlarged and covered with a grayish white thick membrane (pseudo-membrane) and the throat inlet is almost occluded. There is pooling of saliva as well.

2. This is a case of severe infectious mononucleosis.

3. It should be differentiated from diphtheria in which there is a grayish, thick membrane situated at laryngeal level and is closely adherent to the surrounding tissues causing severe life-threatening stridor.

4. Treatment includes:
   a. General measures.
      - Symptomatic relief with paracetamol or NSAIDs.
      - Saline mouthwashes.
      - Antibiotics to prevent super added infection due to bacteria. Ampicillin should be avoided as it causes generalised macular rash. As this patient has obstructive symptoms, a short course of steroids (for 5 days) in tapering dose can be beneficial.
   b. Treatment of complications.
   Hepatitis, myocarditis, encephalitis are treated symptomatically.
   Splenic rupture requires immediate surgery (repeated deep palpation of spleen should be avoided in these cases).

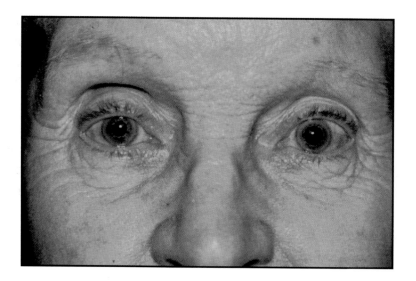

This lady had haemoptysis and clubbing of her fingers.
1. What abnormalities are shown?
2. What is the diagnosis?
3. What is the primary diagnosis?
4. Name few other causes of this abnormality.
5. What do you expect to see in her chest?

ANSWERS

1. The abnormalities shown are:
   a. The right eyelid is drooped (partial ptosis).
   b. The right eye is sunken (enophthalmos).
   c. The right pupil is small in size as compared to the left (meiosis).
2. Right Horner's syndrome. Other features include loss of sweating on the affected side (anhidrosis) and loss of ciliospinal reflex.
3. A Pancoast' tumour in view of the history of smoking, haemoptysis and clubbing seems most likely primary diagnosis.
4. The causes include:
   a. Trauma – injury to cervical sympathetic ganglia.
   b. Post-surgical (iatrogenic).
   c. Wallenberg's syndrome—posterior inferior cerebellar artery (PICA).
   d. Syringomyelia / syringobulbia.
5. The chest X-ray may show a homogeneous opacity in the right upper zone involving apices (Pancoast's tumour). There may or may not be a pulmonary effusion.

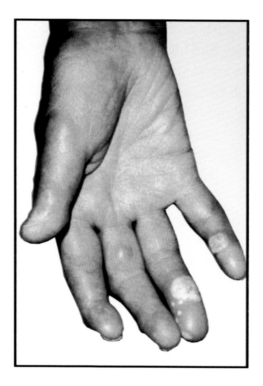

This patient had uncontrolled hypertension. He also consumed three units of whisky a day.

1. What abnormality is shown in this slide?
2. What is the diagnosis?
3. How would you confirm it?
4. What is the treatment?

ANSWERS

1. There are well-circumscribed white/yellow lesions over the palmar side of right ring and little finger. Other digits are also swollen.
2. This is chronic tophaceous gout.
3. Aspiration of the lesion with a needle and looking for negatively birefringent crystals of urate under microscope.
4. The main treatment is to reduce uric acid on long-term basis and keep a serum level <5 mg/dl. Adequate control of blood pressure and use of allopurinol and uricosuric agents on long-term basis achieve this.

   Surgical excision of large tophi gives immediate relief but is rarely required.

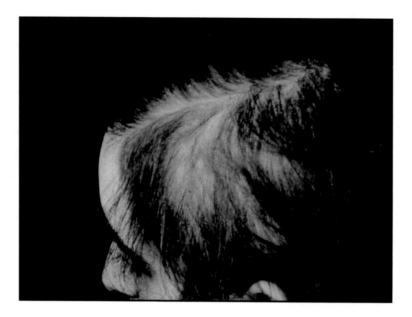

This young woman complained of malaise, painful joints and oral ulcers.

1. What is shown in this slide?
2. What is the primary diagnosis?
3. Classify different types of such abnormality.
4. What other complications this patient might have?

ANSWERS

1. There are areas of scalp without hair called alopecia areata.
2. The primary diagnosis is systemic lupus erythematosus as she has arthralgia and oral ulcers.
3. They are classified as:
   a. Scarring alopecia—due to trauma and chemicals or burns.
   b. Non-scarring alopecia—due to autoimmune disorders, i.e. SLE, secondary syphilis, hyper or hypothyroidism, iron deficiency or pituitary insufficiency.
   c. Androgenic alopecia—commonest form of alopecia in males.
   d. Alopecia totalis—if alopecia involves whole scalp.
   e. Alopecia universalis—if alopecia involves scalp, eyebrows, eyelashes and body hair including axillary and pubic hair.
4. Other complications in this patient will be those of SLE namely:
   a. Lupus nephritis.
   b. Lupus cerebritis.
   c. Pericarditis.
   d. Vasculitis.
   e. Arteriovenous thromboses (Hughe's syndrome).
   f. Haemolytic anaemia.
   g. Purpura.

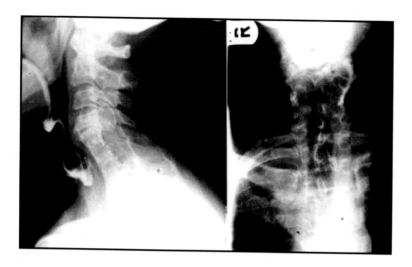

This patient had a short neck and also had difficulty in moving his neck.

1. What is shown in these X-rays?
2. What is the diagnosis?
3. What other associations you know of this abnormality?

ANSWERS

1. The X-ray shows fusion of the lower four cervical vertebrae resulting in short neck. A barium swallow shows indentation of oesophagus due to deformity of the cervical spine.
2. The diagnosis is Klippel-Feil syndrome.
3. The other associations are:
   a. Short neck.
   b. Limited mobility.
   c. Low hairline.
   d. Neurological abnormalities due to platybasia and syringo-myelia.

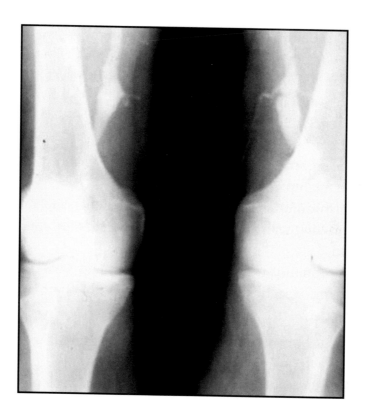

This patient had recurrent ischaemia of his both lower limbs.
1. What is this investigation?
2. What abnormality is shown?
3. Why is this patient getting recurrent ischaemia of his lower limbs?
4. What treatment can be offered?

ANSWERS

1. This is a bilateral popliteal artery angiogram.
2. It shows aneurysms of both popliteal arteries.
3. The aneurysms may contain a clot and recurrent embolization distally results in ischaemia.
4. Aneurysectomy for all asymptomatic aneurysms > 2 cm and for all symptomatic aneurysms regardless of size.

If distal thrombosis is present, catheter directed thrombolysis should be attempted.

If distal thrombosis is absent or recanalised, then saphenous vein by pass grafting with proximal and distal ligation of aneurysms is performed.

In large aneurysms leading to surrounding vessel or nerve compression, resection of aneurysms in addition to grafting is recommended.

NB: Poplitieal aneurysms account for approximately 85% of all peripheral artery aneurysms.

Distal occlusion leads to amputation in up to 30% of patients.

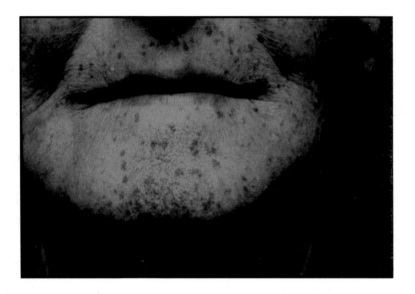

This patient was found to be anaemic. One of his brothers died of massive gastrointestinal bleeding.

1. What abnormality is shown in this slide?
2. What is the diagnosis?
3. How would you confirm it?
4. What treatment is available?

ANSWERS

1. There are multiple 1-2 mm sized, telangiectasias distributed over upper and lower lip, and perioral skin. The skin is also pale.
2. Osler-Weber-Rendu's disease.
3. The diagnosis is made from clinical triad of telangiectasia, haemorrhage and familial pattern. Following may be helpful in the diagnosis:
   - Per laparotomy endoscopic visualization in a dark operating theatre.
   - Video pill to see telangiectasia in the intestinal tract.
4. No definite treatment is available except surgery. However, trial of different agents has not been fruitful.

NB: The condition is simple autosomal dominant trait and affects both sexes equally. The vessels are very delicate and bleed easily due to thin lining of endothelial cells resulting in increased fragility and bleeding. Telangiectasia may be on any part of the skin. These blanch on pressure as blood is not extravasated and is still in the vessels.

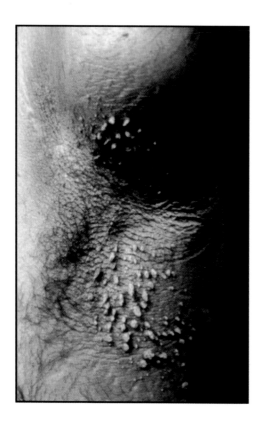

This patient was anaemic, asthenic and anorexic for the last few months.

1. Describe the abnormality.
2. What name is given to it?
3. What is the underlying diagnosis?
4. Name few other causes of this abnormality.

ANSWERS

1. The skin of left axilla shows brown to black hyperpigmentation with multiple confluent papillomas, resulting in velvety elevation of the surface of epidermis.
2. Acanthosis nigricans.
3. Carcinoma of stomach (60%).
4. The other causes include:
   - Idiopathic/congenital obesity.
   - Acquired obesity.
   - Cushing's syndrome.
   - Diabetes mellitus.
   - Acromegaly.
   - Stein-Leventhal syndrome.
   - Adenocarcinoma.
   - Squamous cell carcinoma and lymphoma.

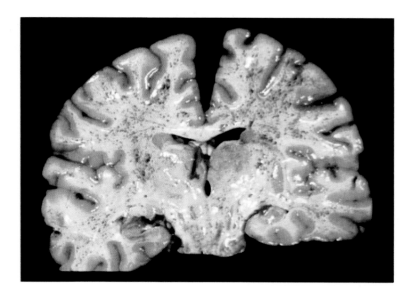

This is postmortem examination of the brain of a man who had a road traffic accident and incurred multiple fractures and injuries.

1. What is shown in this slide?
2. What is the diagnosis?
3. What treatment could be offered?
4. Where else would you see such lesions?

ANSWERS

1. This slide shows a section of brain. There are multiple, minute and widely dispersed micro emboli giving rise to multiple cerebral petechial haemorrhages.
2. Fat embolism.
3. This include:
   - General medical management.
   - Measures directed to restore circulation.
   - Rehabilitation.
4. There may be petechial haemorrhages in the axillae and groins.

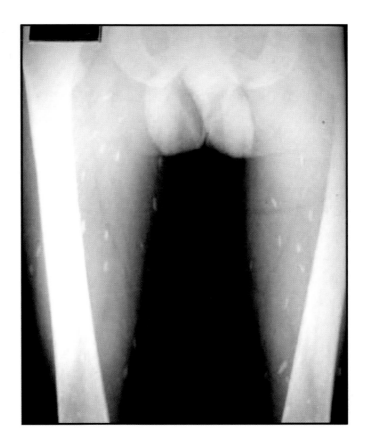

This man complained of pain and discomfort in his thighs.
1. What abnormality do you see in this picture?
2. What is the diagnosis?
3. What is the treatment?

ANSWERS

1. There are multiple elongated hyperdense opacities in the soft tissue of both thighs.
2. Cysticercosis.
3. Praziquantel 50-100 mg/kg/d in three divided doses for two weeks or albendazole 400 mg twice daily with fatty meals from 1-3 weeks are the drugs of choice for cysticercosis. Steroids are given during therapy to avoid reactions.

NB: Cysticercosis occurs after auto-infection or hetero-infection by eggs of *T. solium* and invasion of tissues by intermediate larval form. Three forms are recognized.

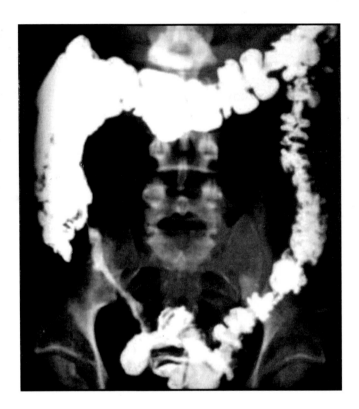

This patient had low grade fever and diarrhoea.

1. What is this investigation?
2. What does it show?
3. What may be the probable diagnosis?
4. What are five radiological features of Crohn's disease?

ANSWERS

1. This is a barium follow through outlining terminal ileum and the part of ascending colon.
2. It shows that the terminal ileum and ileocaecal area is contracted, irregular with distortion of caecum. This is also called string sign of Kantor.
3. The probable diagnosis is Crohn's disease.
4. The five radiological features include:
   - Loss of mucosal details and rigidity of involved segment.
   - Cobble-stoned appearance of mucosa.
   - Stricture-string sign of Kantor.
   - Fistulae.
   - Fibrosis.

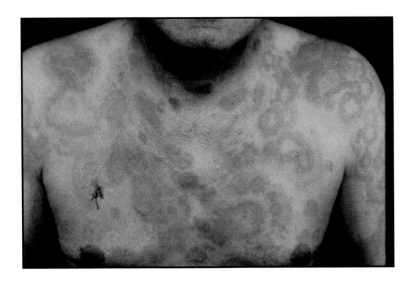

This man was losing weight and developed this generalized rash.

1. Describe the rash.
2. What name is given to it?
3. What may be the underlying pathology?
4. Name few skin markers of internal malignancy.

ANSWERS

1. The slide shows a generalized erythematous rash, circular in shape, with surrounding redness and central pallor. There is also a stitch in the skin from where biopsy had been taken (concentric, arcuate lesions looking like grain of soft wood).
2. Erythema gyratum repens.
3. This is associated with malignant disease and is a useful marker of internal malignancy.

   NB: The rash normally disappears after successful treatment of the malignancy or underlying disease. These usually represent a hypersensitivity reaction to some components of malignant disease.
4. The skin markers of internal malignancies are:
   a. Dermatomyositis.
   b. Acanthosis nigricans.
   c. Migratory thrombophlebitis.
   d. Icthyosis.
   e. Alopecia.
   f. Pruritus.
   g. Clubbing.
   h. Erythema multiforme.
   i. Urticaria.
   j. Dermatitis herpetiformis.
   k. Herpes zoster.
   l. Paget's disease of breast.

SLIDE - 50

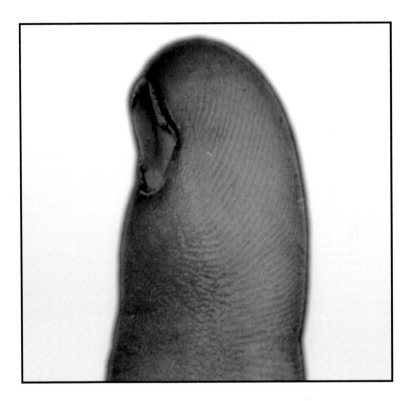

This patient complained of exertional dyspnoea and oedema of feet.

1. What abnormality is shown in this slide?
2. What haematological abnormality would you suspect?
3. Is this abnormality related to any serious condition and if so which one?

ANSWERS

1. This shows concavity in the nail plate called koilonychia.
2. Iron deficiency anaemia.
3. Yes.

   Plummer-Vinson's or Patterson Brown Kelly's syndrome which is characterized by iron deficiency anaemia, oesophageal webs and postcricoid carcinoma of the oesophagus.

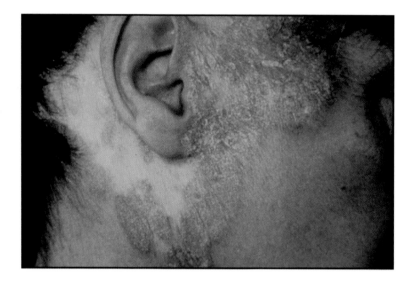

This patient had this progressive rash for many months.
1. Describe the rash.
2. What other abnormalities do you see?
3. What is the most likely diagnosis?
4. How would you confirm it clinically?

ANSWERS

1. There is an indurated, scaly, progressive rash involving the front of pinna, zygomatic area and upper part of the neck.
2. There is scarring behind the ear and alopecia called scarring alopecia.
3. Lupus vulgaris.
4. Clinically if the border of lesion in pressed with a glass slide, the underlying skin appears as an apple jelly.

   However, the diagnosis is confirmed histologically.

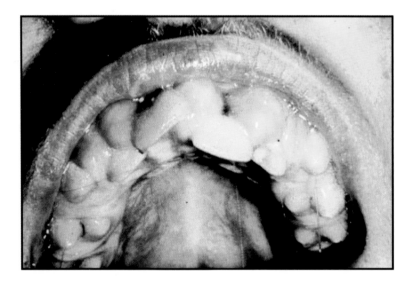

This slide is from an epileptic and mentally retarded patient.
1. What abnormality do you see?
2. What is the cause?
3. Give few other causes of this abnormality.

ANSWERS

1. There is hypertrophy of the gums and mal-alignment of the teeth.
2. This appearance is due to phenytoin toxicity as this patient was on phenytoin for control of his epilepsy.
3. The gingival hypertrophy can occur in:
   a. Myelomonocytic leukaemia.
   b. Cyclosporin toxicity.
   c. Gingivitis.
   d. Pregnancy.
   e. Idiopathic familial fibromatosis.

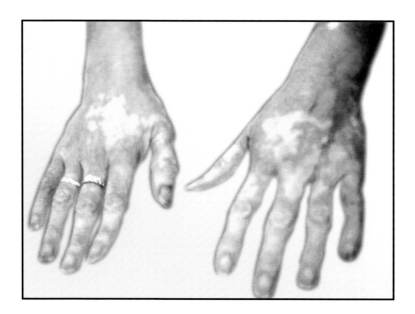

This is a diabetic patient.

1. Describe the abnormality.
2. What name is given to it?
3. Name few other associated conditions.

ANSWERS

1. There are symmetrical patches of depigmentation on the dorsum of both hands and digits with surrounding normal pigmented skin.
2. This is called vitiligo.
3. The associated conditions are:
   - Diabetes mellitus.
   - Hypothyroidism.
   - Hyperthyroidism.
   - Pernicious anaemia.
   - Addison's disease.
   - Hypoparathyroidism.
   - Myasthenia gravis.
   - Alopecia areata.
   - Morphoea and lichen sclerosis.
   - Halo naevus.
   - Malignant melanoma.

SLIDE - 54

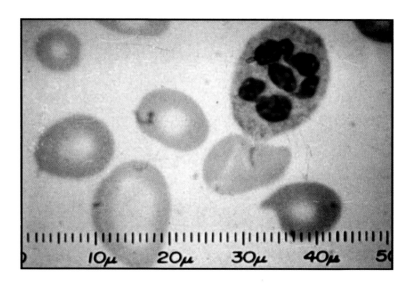

This is a slide of peripheral film of a patient who complained of lassitude, anorexia and clinically had pallor and swollen feet.

1. What abnormalities are shown in this slide?
2. What is the primary diagnosis?
3. How would you confirm it?
4. What is the treatment?

ANSWERS

1. This slide shows that the size of RBC's is enlarged (diameter $> 7\,\mu$) called macrocytes (megaloblasts if from the bone marrow) or macro-ovalocytes, and the neutrophils shows more than 5 lobes called hypersegmented polymorphonuclear leukocyte.

2. Pernicious anaemia, B_{12} deficiency anaemia.

3. Following help to confirm the diagnosis:
   a. MCV between 110 and 120 fl.
   b. Bone marrow shows erythroid hyperplasia with megaloblastic changes.
   c. Raised LDH and bilirubin.
   d. Reduced B_{12} levels < 100 pg/ml.
   e. Four-staged Schilling's test to document decreased absorption of vitamin B_{12}.

4. The treatment is with intramuscular injection of $100\,\mu g$ of vitamin B_{12} daily for one week, then weekly for one month then monthly at three monthly intervals for the rest of life.

   Hypokalaemia occurs and should be treated. Other haematinics including iron and folate should also be supplemented after replacement with vitamin B_{12}.

NB:

Schilling's test

It is done in four stages.

   i. *First stage:* 1 mg of B_{12} is given im to saturate plasma transport proteins. Radiolabelled vitamin B_{12} (^{61}Co) is administered orally and 24 hours urinary collection is performed. Normal excretion is > 7 % of the dose where as with impaired absorption it will be $< 3\%$.

   ii. *Second stage:* Radiolabelled B_{12} is given with intrinsic factor. If pernicious anaemia (a lack of intrinsic factor) is the cause of vitamin B_{12} deficiency, this combination should correct the absorption abnormality.

   iii. *Third stage:* If still $< 3\%$ excretion then consider problems/ diseases of the terminal ileum or blind loop syndrome, pancreatic enzyme deficiency or fish tape worm infestation.

   iv. *Fourth stage:* The test is repeated after correction of terminal ileum disease, or after a course of antibiotics in case of bacterial over growth in blind loop syndrome, or replacement of pancreatic enzymes and after treatment of tape worm (Diphyllobothrium cephalus latum) infestation. The excretion in urine is measured again and it should improve to $> 7\%$.

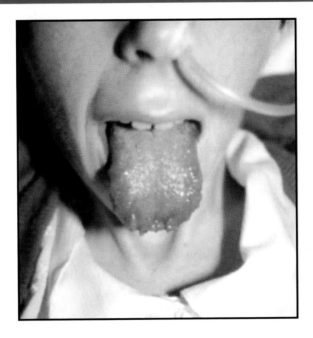

This patient was pregnant and had paroxysmal hypertension, pallor and palpitations.

1. What abnormalities are shown in this picture?
2. What is the name given to lesions at the tip of the tongue?
3. Why is this patient hypertensive?
4. What are associated conditions?
5. What is the diagnosis?

ANSWERS

1. There are multiple nodular swellings of 5 mm size on the tip of the tongue. A nasogastric tube is also inserted.
2. These are called mucosal neuromas.
3. There was a pheochromocytoma in this patient causing paroxysmal hypertension.
4. The associated conditions include:
   • Calcitonin-secreting tumours (medullary thyroid carcinoma and hyperparathyroidism – type 2 MEN.
   • Medullary thyroid carcinoma, multiple mucosal neuromas, marfanoid features- type 2b MEN.
   • Neurofibromatosis (von Recklinghausen's disease) and islet cell tumours (rare).
   • von Hippel-Lindau disease, pancreatic cysts, renal cysts, adenomas and carcinomas.
5. In this case diagnosis is type 2b MEN also called type 3 MEN.

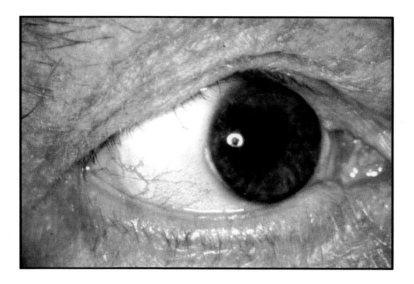

This 65-year-old patient had aches and pains in his bones for the last one year. He was found to be dehydrated and semi-comatosed. He had multiple fractures of his ribs and X-ray of the skull was also abnormal.

1. What is the abnormality?
2. What is it?
3. What is it due to?
4. What is the primary diagnosis?
5. How would you confirm it?

ANSWERS

1. There is a white crescentic line on the corneoscleral junction (limbus) of right eye.
2. This is corneal calcification.
3. It is due to hypercalcaemia.
4. Multiple myeloma, the skull X-ray is showing multiple punched out lesions.
5. Multiple myeloma is confirmed by the followings:

   Multiple punched out lytic lesions in the skull, ribs, long bones, and pelvis on skeletal survey.

   Monoclonal gammopathy with suppression of other immunoglobulins on immune electrophoresis.

   Presence of plasma cells (>10-100%) in bone marrow.

   If two out of above three are present, multiple myeloma is strongly suspected.

   NB: The incidence of IgG myeloma is 60%, IgA 25% and light chain 15%.

   Other laboratory findings include:

   Anaemia, Bence Jones proteins in the urine, hypercalcaemia (cause for dehydration and semi-comatosed state in this patient), raised ESR, phosphaturia, glycosuria and uricosuria.

   The white crescent due to hypercalcaemia should be differentiated from age-related arcus (arcus senilis). The crescent due to hypercalcaemia occurs at the limbus, at 3 and 9'O clock position and is static and disappears after correction of hypercalcaemia.

   The crescent due to age-related arcus occurs in the cornea at the periphery and there is a clear rim from the limbus. It occurs at 6 and 12'O clock position and is progressive in nature and indicates underlying hypercholesterolaemia. It is permanent.

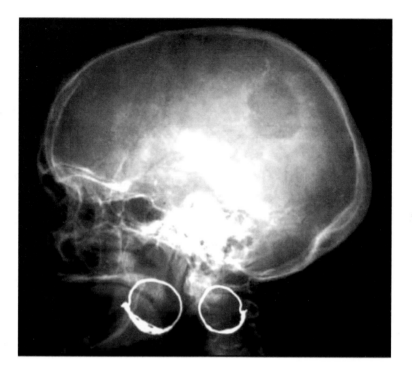

This patient presented with dysphagia and a swelling in front of neck.

1. What abnormality is seen here?
2. What is the diagnosis?
3. What is the differential diagnosis?

ANSWERS

1. There is a large osteolytic lesion on the parieto-occipital area of the skull.
2. This is a metastatic deposit from a thyroid carcinoma as this patient has dysphagia and goitre which may probably be malignant.
3. The differential diagnosis of lytic lesions in the skull include:
   i. Metastases from cancer of pancreas, stomach, kidney, heart, and ovary.
   ii. Multiple myeloma.
   iii. Hyperparathyroidism.
   iv. Hand-Schüller-Christian disease.
   v. Histiocytosis-X.

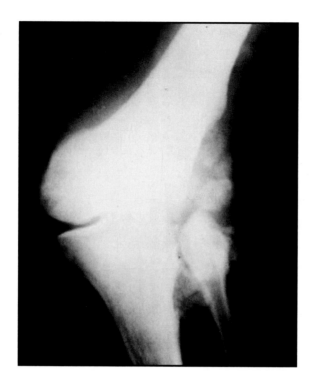

This picture is from a patient who had diabetes mellitus.
1. What is this?
2. What does it show?
3. What is the diagnosis?
4. Name few other differential diagnoses.

ANSWERS

1. This is a radiograph of left knee joint.
2. It shows loss of joint space due to destruction of the articular cartilage and mal-alignment of the bones around knee joint.
3. Charcot's joint or neuropathic joint. They can lead to arthritis mutilans.
4. The causes of neuropathic joints are:
    i. Tabes dorsalis.
    ii. Diabetes mellitus.
    iii. Syringomyelia.
    iv. Spinal cord injury.
    v. Sub-acute combined degeneration of cord.
    vi. Leprosy.
    vii. Peripheral nerve injury.

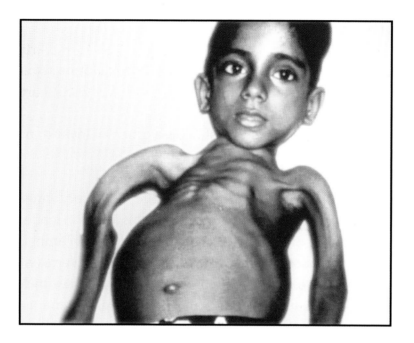

This slide is of a nine-year-old boy.

1. Describe the abnormalities.
2. What is the underlying metabolic abnormality?
3. What is the diagnosis?

ANSWERS

1. The abnormalities are:
   i. Thin formed skull
   ii. Widened epiphysis of humrus leading to deformity of bones, i.e. bowing of the limbs.
   iii. Rickety rosary.
   iv. Grooves in the subcostal area due to inward pull of diaphragm.
2. Rickets.
3. It is due to vitamin D deficiency due to dietary causes or inadequate sunlight or malabsorption. This results in inadequate mineralization of bone matrix. Hydroxylation of vitamin D and its active metabolite, i.e. 1,25 dihydroxy cholecalciferol (vitamin D_3) is defective or inadequate due to many causes including renal causes, e.g. Fanconi's syndrome (proximal renal tubular acidosis Type-2 RTA), chronic renal failure, renal osteodystrophy, dialysis induced bone disease and distal renal tubular acidosis (Type-1 RTA). Other causes include multiple myeloma, X-linked hypophosphataemia and mesenchymal tumours.

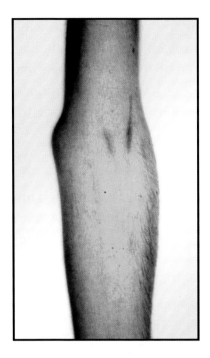

This drug addict was brought to accident and emergency department with weight loss, high grade fever and anaemia.He had a pre-cordial murmur and swelling in the left hypochondrium.

1. What is shown in this slide?
2. What is the diagnosis?
3. What is the treatment?
4. Is this patient left handed?

ANSWERS

1. There are linear marks on the left ante-cubital fossa.
2. The diagnosis is infective endocarditis due to main line drug abuse as evidenced by thrombophlebitis (linear marks) over the left ante-cubital fossa, low grade fever, anaemia and a precordial murmur. The swelling in left hypochondrium is due to splenomegaly.
3. Intravenous antibiotics.

    In drug addicts *S. aureus* accounts for 60%, streptococci and enterococci, 50%, gram-ve bacilli, fungi and unusual organisms are also involved. Other organisms like *S. epidermidis*, histoplasma, brucella, candida and aspergillus are also common in intravenous drug abusers.

    For staphylococci, which are methicillin resistant following antibiotics may be used:

Nafcillin	1.5 g IV 4 hourly for 4-6 weeks
Oxacillin	1.5 g IV 4 hourly for 4-6 weeks
Cefazolin	2 g IV 8 hourly
Vancomycin	15 mg/ kg IV 12 hourly
Aminoglycosides	1 mg/ kg IV 8 hourly for 5 days initially then continued for 2 weeks

    Antifungal agents are used if fungi are isolated.
4. No, this patient is right handed. The arm shown is the left arm and only a right handed person can inject drugs in left arm with his right hand which is dominant, and *vice versa*.

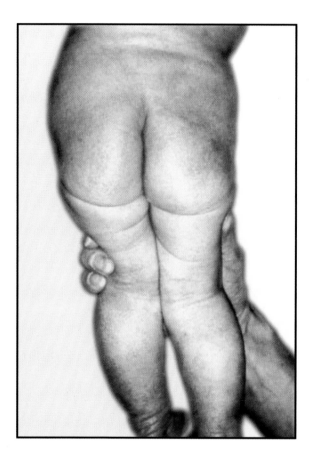

This young boy was brought to accident and emergency department with upper respiratory tract infection.

1. Describe the abnormality.
2. What is the diagnosis?
3. What is the differential diagnosis?
4. What name is given to this abnormality?

ANSWERS

1. The gluteal region shows bluish macular area without any scales or ulceration in a healthy looking boy.
2. Mongolian blue spot.
3. It should he differentiated from battered baby syndrome.
4. Not significant.

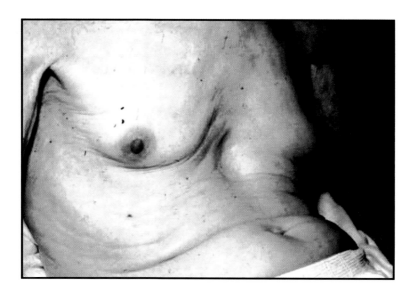

This picture is of a 65-year-old man.
1. What abnormality is shown here?
2. Name five drugs which can cause this abnormality.
3. What other three conditions can lead to this abnormality?

ANSWERS

1. This slide shows prominent breasts in a male patient called gynaecomastia.
2. The five drugs are:
   a. Spironolactone.
   b. Cimetidine.
   c. Digoxin.
   d. Methyldopa.
   e. Oestrogen preparation.
3. The other three conditions leading to this abnormality are:
   a. Chronic liver disease.
   b. Klinefelter's syndrome.
   c. Bronchogenic carcinoma.

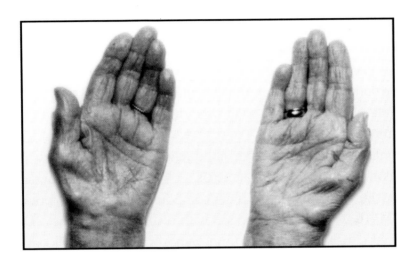

This 76-year-old lady fell down on the ground with outstretched hands.

1. What abnormality is shown?
2. What may have caused this abnormality?
3. What is the diagnosis?
4. How would you confirm it?
5. Name few other causes of this abnormality.

ANSWERS

1. There is wasting of muscles leading to guttering of the outer half of thenar eminences of both hands.
2. This patient suffered from bilateral Colle's fracture and was mismanaged in plaster, thus resulting in this deformity.
3. Bilateral carpal tunnel syndrome due to bilateral median nerve compression.
4. Confirmation is by nerve conduction studies. Sensory nerve action potential (SNAP) latency is prolonged with slow conduction velocity. It is compared to ulnar compound motor action potentials (CMAP) which are prolonged with distal motor latency (DML).
5. Other causes of Corpal Tunnel Syndrome include following:
   a. Musculoskeletal disorders, e.g. cysts, ganglions in wrist area compressing on median nerve.
   b. Rheumatoid arthritis.
   c. Endocrine causes include diabetic mellitus, hypothyroidism, acromegaly, pregnancy.
   d. Miscellaneous causes include leukaemia, multiple myeloma, amyloidosis, sarcoidosis, Paget's disease.

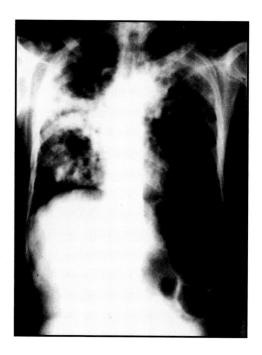

This patient presented to the accident and emergency department with chronic history of cough, fever and sudden onset of severe abdominal pain. On examination, he was pyrexial and drowsy with tender abdomen.

1. Describe abnormalities on this slide.
2. What has the patient developed?
3. What is the primary diagnosis?

ANSWERS

1. This plain radiograph includes both chest and upper two-thirds of abdomen. There are soft tissue shadows of different density in both left upper and right middle and lower zones. There is a fine crescent of air under the right dome of the diaphragm.
2. This patient has developed acute peritonitis due to perforation of a hollow viscus.
3. The primary diagnosis is pulmonary tuberculosis leading to ileocaecal tuberculosis resulting in perforation thus causing acute peritonitis.

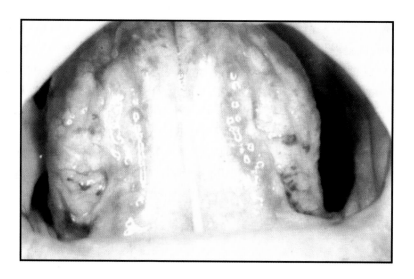

This patient had marked pallor.
1. What abnormalities are shown in this slide?
2. What is the diagnosis?
3. Why is this patient anaemic?
4. Is family history important?

ANSWERS

1. The under surface of the tongue shows clusters of tiny blood vessels and marked pallor of frenulum linguae and ventral aspect of tongue.
2. Hereditary haemorrhagic telangiectasia.
3. These telangiectasia are present throughout the gastrointestinal tract and continuously bleed, thus resulting in acute or chronic blood loss causing severe anaemia.
4. Yes. The other family members may have the same problem, which is an autosomal dominant trait. It is also called Osler-Weber-Rendu disease.

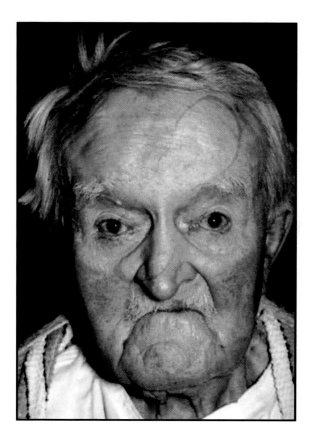

This 73-year-old man had left swollen thigh and heart failure.
1. What is abnormal on this slide?
2. What is the diagnosis?
3. How are these two presenting ailments related?
4. What biochemical markers you know of this primary diagnosis?

ANSWERS

1. There is asymmetry of the skull. The right temporoparietal area is bulging. There is some malar redness.
2. This is a classical face of Paget's disease.
3. Paget's disease of bone can lead to bone deformities and high cardiac output failure due to A-V fistulae in bone matrix. Both were present in this case.
4. The biochemical markers include:
   a. Raised alkaline phosphatase.
   b. Raised excretion of urinary hydroxyproline.
   c. Osteocalcin.
   d. PICP.
   e. TRAP (Tartaric resistant acid phosphatase).
   f. Urinary hydroxy lysin.
   g. Urinary deoxypyridinoline, N-telopeptide and C-telopeptide.

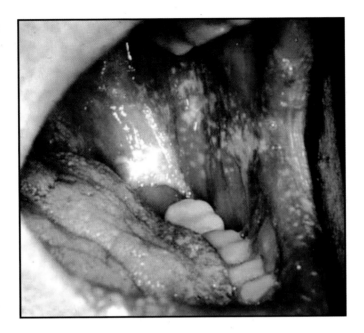

This patient had soreness in his mouth.

1. What abnormality is visible?
2. What is the diagnosis?
3. What is the treatment?

ANSWERS

1. There are grayish white linear, lacy and polygonal areas on the inner side of left cheek. Few lesions are seen on the tongue as well.
2. Lichen planus of the oral mucosa.
3. The treatment consists of topical steroids in the form of creams or lotions. Tretinoin cream 0.05% to lesions is also used with good results. Topical tacrolimus is also effective. Systemic steroids may be useful in severe form of the disease. Cyclosporine can also be used.

SLIDE - 68

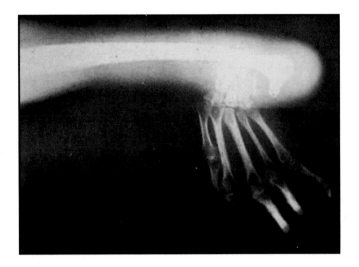

This patient had difficulty in holding objects in his hands.
1. What abnormalities do you see in this slide?
2. What name is given to this abnormality?
3. What might have caused this abnormality?

ANSWERS

1. This radiograph shows that the humerus is deformed at the lower end, there is absence of ulna and radius, the carpus, metacarpus and phalanges are also deformed.
2. Phocomelia.
3. Thalidomide – which was used in 60's for controlling hyperemesis gravidarum.

NB: Thalidomide has re-emerged and it is used now in different condition, e.g. aphthous ulcers, erythema nodosum leprosum, discoid lupus, lupus erythematosus, myeloma and various cancerous conditions. It is important that this drug should be used in non-pregnant patients only.

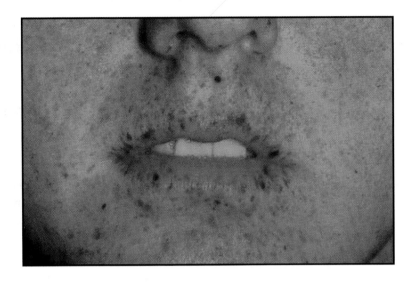

This patient had abdominal pain and passed blood in the stools.
1. What is the abnormality?
2. What is the diagnosis?
3. How are these symptoms explained?
4. What are the complications?

ANSWERS

1. There are diffuse dark brown pigmented macules at the tips and mucocutaneous junction and the mouth. Few are also present on the skin of chin and around nose.
2. Peutz-Jeghers syndrome (P-J syndrome).
3. This syndrome is characterized by hamartomata including polyps in the small bowel. This can lead to intestinal obstruction and bleeding due to ulceration.
4. Complications of P-J syndrome include.
   • Intestinal obstruction.
   • Intussusception.
   • Gastrointestinal bleeding.
   • Gastrointestinal malignancies.
   • Association with non-gastrointestinal malignancies, e.g. breast, nasal cavity, cervix, uterus, ovaries and testicles.
   • Hypokalaemia.

SLIDE - 70

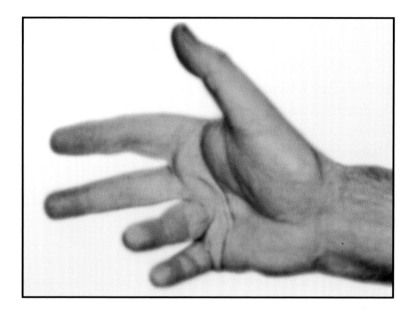

1. What is shown in this picture?
2. Mention few causes of this deformity.
3. What is the mode of inheritance?

ANSWERS

1. There is flexion of the ring and little fingers of the right hand, with puckering of the skin at their bases. The transverse creases are narrowed at that point as well. This is Dupuytren's contracture.
2. This deformity is associated with:
   a. Idiopathic causes.
   b. Traumatic, especially due to vibrating tools.
   c. Diabetes mellitus.
   d. Chronic liver disease.
   e. Use of antiepileptics especially phenytoin.
3. Autosomal dominant.

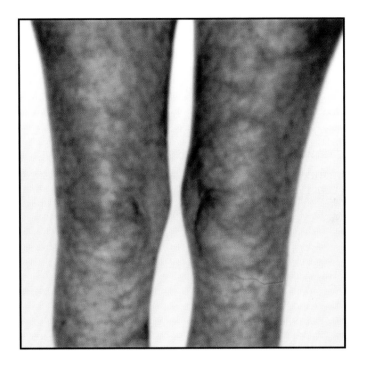

1. Describe the abnormality.
2. What name is given to this?
3. What are the causes of this abnormality?

ANSWERS

1. There is mottled, lacy, reticular pattern on both thighs and shins with central pallor.
2. Livedo reticularis.
3. This abnormality is associated with:
   - Polyarteritis nodosa.
   - Atherosclerotic microemboli.
   - Systemic lupus erythematosus.
   - Antiphospholipid antibody syndrome (Hughes syndrome).
   - Occult malignancy.

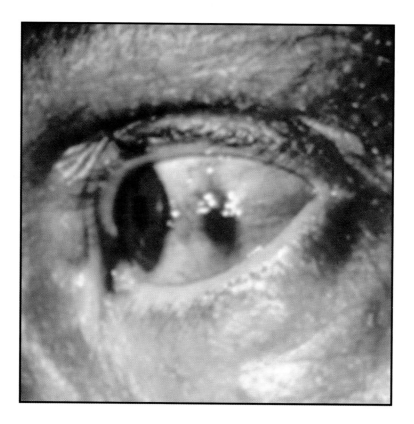

This man had painful joints and noticed that the colour of his urine becomes dark after sometime.

1. What is shown in this picture?
2. What is the diagnosis?
3. What is the metabolic abnormality?

ANSWERS

1. There is dark brown discolouration of sclera on the lateral aspect of left eye, at the insertion of lateral rectus muscle.
2. Ochronosis—the triad consists of arthritis, ochronotic pigmentation and urine which darkens on standing.
3. Alcaptonuria—It is an autosomal recessive disease. The genetic defect is due to deficiency of an enzyme called homogentisic acid oxidase which leads to excessive accumulation of homogentisic acid which is a normal intermediate product in the metabolism of phenylalanine and tyrosine.

NB: This is an autosomal recessive disorder with a frequency of 1in 200,000 births. The triad is already mentioned. On treatment with strong alkali, the urine darkens. On treatment with ferric chloride, urine turns purple-black in colour.

Chemical tests, chromatographic characteristics or specific enzyme assay also confirms it. Treatment includes ascorbic acid as a strong reducing agent along with symptomatic treatment of osteoarthritis.

SLIDE - 73

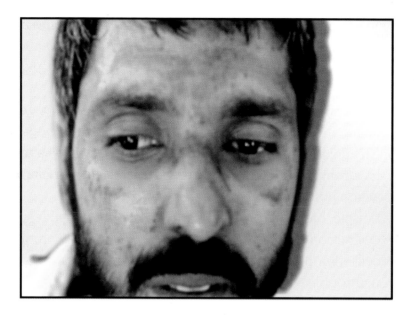

This picture is of a man with history of smoking that presented with breathlessness and haemoptysis.

1. What abnormality is shown in this picture?
2. What name is given to this abnormal sign?
3. What is the diagnosis?
4. Name three diagnostic tests.

ANSWERS

1. There is violaceous discolouration around the eyes, cheeks and the bridge of nose with few telangiectatic areas present over the forehead.
2. Heliotrope rash.
3. Dermatomyositis.
4. The three diagnostic tests are:
    i. Creatinine kinase is markedly elevated along with 5′-aldolase.
    ii. Electromyography (EMG) reveals polyphasic or multiphasic action potentials.
    iii. Muscle biopsy from affected muscle shows widespread destruction of muscles and infiltration of chronic inflammatory cells (lymphocytes, monocytes, plasma cells and rarely neutrophils). There are some regenerating fibres as well.

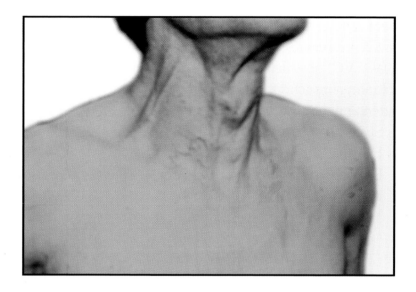

This man smoked sixty cigarettes per day and had breathlessness and giddy spells.

1. What abnormal sign is shown here?
2. What may be the underlying cause?
3. What is the treatment?

ANSWERS

1. There are engorged jugular veins in the neck. Few dilated vessels are also present on the front of upper chest. This is superior vena caval (SVC) obstruction.
2. Infiltrating bronchogenic carcinoma.
3. The treatment include:
    i. Systemic steroids.
    ii. External beam radiation.
    iii. Endovascular stenting unless concomitant tumour resection is planned.

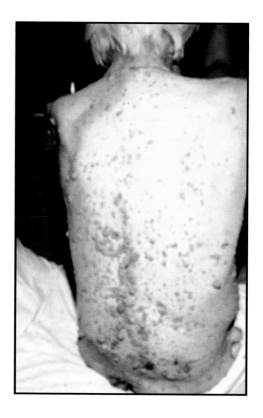

This 58-year-old man had headache and paroxysmal hypertension.

1. What is the abnormality?
2. What is the diagnosis?
3. How do you explain his hypertension and headaches?
4. What is the inheritance?

ANSWERS

1. There are multiple, nodular swellings over the back of this patient. Few are sessile and a couple of them are pedunculated.
2. Multiple neurofibromatosis or von Recklinghausen's disease.
3. Neurofibromatosis is associated with intracranial tumours like meningioma, gliomas or acoustic neuroma and pheochromocytoma. The first three can explain headache and the last one paroxysmal hypertension.
4. Autosomal dominant.

NB: Neurofibromatosis can be divided into 8-varieties but four are more common. Out of these four, two are most common, i.e. type I or peripheral and type 2 or central.

The other two are segmental neurofibromatosis and plexiform neurofibromatosis.

The gene of type I is localized on chromosome 17 and for type 2 on chromosome 22.

Axillary freckling is the pathognomonic sign of neurofibromatosis.

Café-au-lait spots or patches are pale brown macules which are 1-20 cm in diameter. They are also common in normal population but more than 5 are abnormal. Associated abnormalities include the following:

   i. Scoliosis.
   ii. Orbital haemangiomas.
   iii. Local gigantism of limbs (plexiform).
   iv. Pheochromocytoma and ganglioneuroma.
   v. Renal artery stenosis.
   vi. Obstructive cardiomyopathy.
   vii. Fibrous dysplasia of bones.
   viii. Lisch's nodules in the iris.

Treatment is surgery essentially for cosmetic reasons. However, tumours causing pressure within the nervous system require excision including pheochromocytoma, if this is feasible.

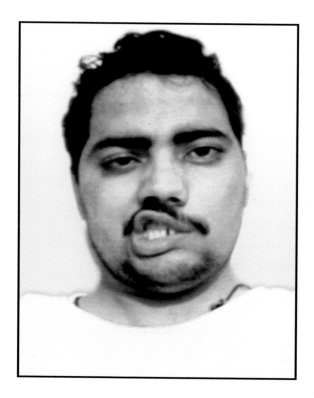

This man complained some discomfort behind his left ear.
1. What abnormalities do you see in this picture?
2. What is the diagnosis?
3. List few causes of this disease.

ANSWERS

1. The angle of mouth is deviated towards the right side.
   There is prominent right nasolabial fold.
2. This patient has left sided Bell's palsy. (He should be asked to wrinkle his forehead, close his eyes, should try to whistle and blow his mouth).
3. The causes of Bell's palsy are numerous including the followings:
   i. Idiopathic.
   ii. Viral infections, i.e. herpes of geniculate ganglion leading to Ramsay Hunt syndrome.
   iii. Acoustic neuroma.
   iv. Guillain-Barré syndrome.
   v. Sarcoidosis (Heerfordt's syndrome).
   vi. Infectious mononucleosis.
   vii. Mononeuritis multiplex.

Melkersson's syndrome, which is rare and consists of recurrent facial paralysis which ultimately becomes permanent, facial (particularly labial) oedema and less constantly, plication of the tongue. Its cause is unknown.

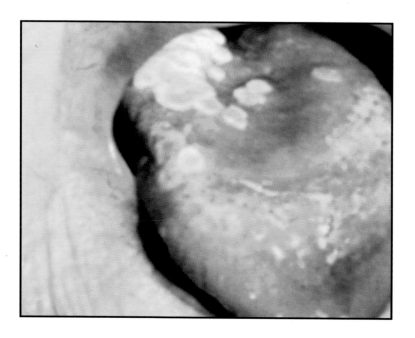

This patient complained of severe burning in his mouth.
1. Describe the abnormality.
2. What is the diagnosis?
3. What treatment would you offer?

ANSWERS

1. There are multiple, circular, raised, lesions covered with white slough. They are in clusters and a few are isolated. Most of them are on the right side of tongue. The tongue is also coated.
2. Herpes zoster of the tongue.
3. Local and systemic acyclovir 800 mg 5 times a day for 5 days.

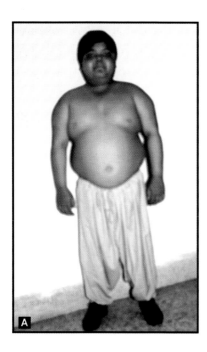 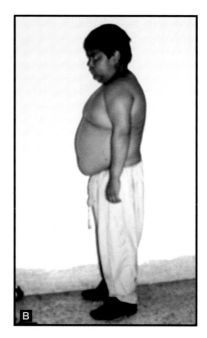

This boy had recurrent sore throat which led to some kidney problem for which he received some treatment.

1. What abnormalities are shown in this picture?
2. What is the primary diagnosis?
3. How can you prevent the complications related to this treatment?

ANSWERS

1. This is a slide of boy from front and side. It shows abnormal distribution of fat, moon-shaped face and swelling over the neck.
2. Cushing's syndrome—In this case it is iatrogenic (patient had post-streptococcal glomerulonephritis for which he received steroids for the treatment of nephritic syndrome which is a well-known complication of streptococcal sore throat).
3. The complications of steroids are numerous but the following are more important:
    i. Diabetes mellitus.
    ii. Osteoporosis.
    iii. Acute psychiatric problems, both dysphoria and euphoria.
    iv. Proximal myopathy.
    v. Acid peptic disease.
    vi. Suppression of growing children.
    vii. Immunosuppression.
    viii. Hepatic enzyme induction.
    ix. Hypokalaemia.

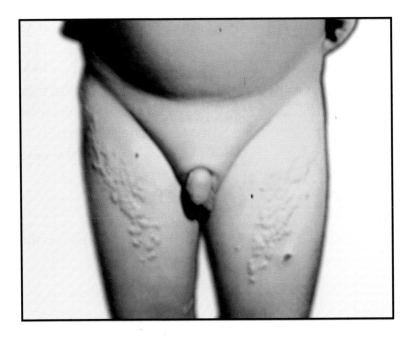

This patient had non-itchy lesions and some abnormality was found on gross inspection of his blood sample.

1. What is the abnormality?
2. Where else would you inspect?
3. What is the treatment?

ANSWERS

1. There are multiple, yellow coloured, papular lesions on front of both thighs.
2. They may also be present on the buttocks and in front of knees.
3. Cholesterol lowering agents, e.g. statins and antihypertriglyceri-demic agents help reducing the size and number of these lesions. Surgical removal is also advised for cosmetic purpose.

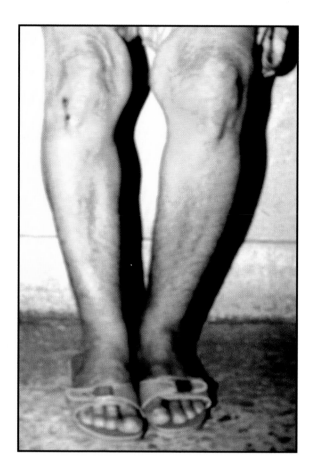

This 76-year-old lady is hard of hearing. She also complained of pain in her left thigh.

1. What abnormality is shown?
2. What may be the diagnosis?
3. Mention few complications of this disease.

ANSWERS

1. The legs are bowed and curved laterally.
2. Paget's disease of bones.
3. Complications include:
   i. Bone deformity.
   ii. Pathological fractures.
   iii. High cardiac output failure
   iv. Entrapment neuropathy of vestibulo-chochlear, facial, optic nerve and platybasia causing pressure effect on upper part of spinal cord.
   v. Osteogenic sarcoma (1%).

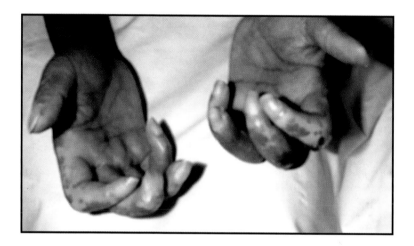

This patient complained of pain and tingling in her hands, especially in the winter season.

1. What abnormality is shown in this picture?
2. What is the name given to this phenomenon?
3. What is the management?

ANSWERS

1. The skin is shiny, tight with areas of pallor of the fingers and palms.
2. Raynaud's phenomenon.
3. Management includes:

General measures

    i. Avoid exposure to cold.
    ii. Wear thermal gloves.
    iii. Avoid trauma.
    iv. Smoke cessation.
    v. Application of emollient on skin.
    vi. Oral beta-blockers and ergot alkaloids should be avoided.

Vasodilators

    i. Low dose nifedipine sustained release 30 mg daily orally.
    ii. Topical or oral nitroglycerine.
    iii. Selective serotonin reuptake inhibitors (SSRI), e.g. fluoxetine 20 mg daily is also effective.
    iv. Aspirin in low dose.

Surgery

    i. Bypass for severe Raynaud's phenomenon.
    ii. Sympathectomy.

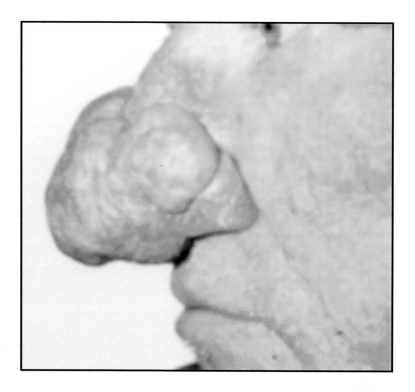

This patient had difficulty in breathing through his nose.
1. What name is given to this abnormality?
2. What are the associated causes?
3. What is the management?

ANSWERS

1. The soft tissue on the tip of the nose is hypertrophied leading to gross deformity and obstruction of the nostrils. It is called rhinophyma.
2. It is associated with rosacea.
3. This condition only responds to surgical reconstruction.

NB: Rosacea is a chronic facial disorder of middle aged and old people. There is a vascular component including erythema and telangiectasia and a tendency to flush easily.

An acneiform component including papules and pustules may also be present. It is the glandular component accompanied by hyperplasia of the soft tissue of the nose and sebaceous hyperplasia which result in rhinophyma. The treatment of rosacea is topical metronidazole gel or cream.

Topical clindamycin twice daily in effective as well.

Erythromycin and tetracycline in doses of 250-500 mg twice daily are also effective but require treatment for 8 weeks.

Minocycline 50-100 mg daily may work in refractory cases.

Isotretinoin may also be helpful. The dose is 0.5-1 mg/ kg/ day orally for 12-28 weeks.

Metronidazole 200 mg twice daily for 3 weeks can also be used.

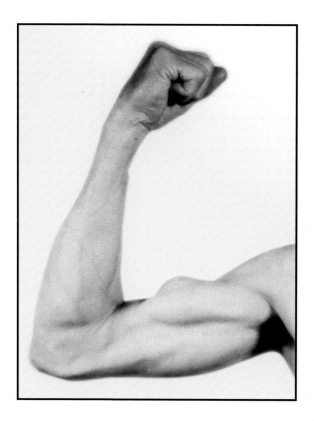

This manual worker was lifting up a heavy object and soon after complained of painful movements of his right upper limb.

1. Describe the abnormality.
2. What may have happened?
3. What is the treatment?

ANSWERS

1. There is subcutaneous rounded swelling over the biceps area of right arm.
2. Rupture of the tendon of long head of the biceps.
3. Surgical repair and re-attachment of the tendon of the long head of biceps to the periosteum is required.

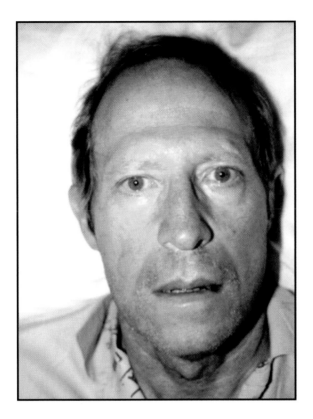

This patient developed Guillain-Barré syndrome and was asked to smile.

1. What abnormality do you see?
2. What complications he has developed?
3. What other clinical tests would you do to confirm this abnormality?
4. How do you grade the severity of Guillain-Barré syndrome?

ANSWERS

1. The patient is unable to give a smile although he is trying. There is a thin film of tears over the lower eyelid.
2. Bilateral facial palsy of lower motor neuron.
3. Ask the patient to close the eyes, the eyeballs roll up (Bell's phenomenon), ask the patient to wrinkle forehead, patient is unable to do that. Patient cannot whistle or blow the mouth.
4. The grading of GB syndrome is as follows:

Grade 0-	Patient is normal.
Grade 1-	Patient can walk unaided for five meters.
Grade 2-	Patient can walk with stick for five meters.
Grade 3-	Patient is chair bound.
Grade 4-	Patient is bed bound.
Grade 5-	Patient is on ventilatory support.
Grade 6-	Patient is dead.

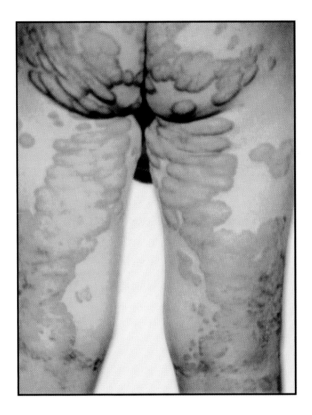

This patient complained of angina on slight exertion.
1. What abnormality has been shown in the picture?
2. Where else do you see this abnormality?
3. What is the relation with angina?
4. What is the treatment?

ANSWERS

1. There are multiple, papular, yellowish brown and well circum-scribed lesions over the buttocks and back of thighs. These are eruptive xanthomas.
2. These are seen on front of thighs, front of knees and elbows and tendo Achilles.
3. These are associated with hyperlipidaemia (familial hypercholes-terolaemia) or combined hypercholesterolaemia and hypertrigly-ceridaemia. These conditions are associated with coronary heart disease.
4. The mainstay of treatment is administration of lipid lowering agents.

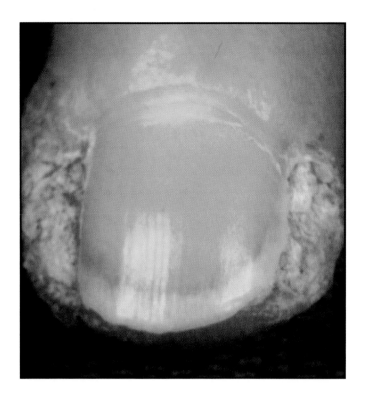

Look at this slide.
1. What is the abnormality?
2. What is the diagnosis?
3. What is the treatment?

ANSWERS

1. The periungual area of the finger is hyperkeratotic, fissured and roughened.
2. Periungual warts.
3. The treatment includes:
   - i. Liquid nitrogen.
   - ii. Keratolytic agents.
   - iii. Podophyllin resin.
   - iv. Imiquimod.
   - v. Surgical removal.
   - vi. Laser therapy.
   - vii. Immunotherapy.
   - viii. Retinoids.

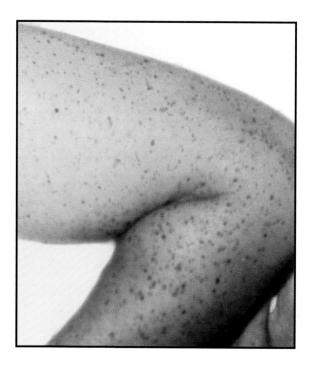

This patient developed bleeding from gums after a pyrexial illness.
1. What abnormality is shown?
2. What may be the diagnosis?
3. What is the treatment?

ANSWERS

1. There a multiple, petechiae of variable sizes ranging from 1 to 2 mm in diameter over the upper arm and forearm.
2. Idiopathic thrombocytopenic purpura.
3. The treatment includes:
    i. Corticosteroids in doses of 1-2 mg/ kg / day until the platelet count is normal.
    ii. High dose intravenous immunoglobulins (IV Ig) 400 mg/ kg/ day for three to five days.
    iii. Splenectomy.
    iv. Danazol 600 mg/ day if patient fails to respond to splenectomy and prednisolone.
    v. Immunosuppressive agents, e.g. azathioprin, vincristine, vin blastine, cyclosporin and cyclophosphamide.
    vi. The role of platelet transfusions is not very promising as the patients have same survival.
    vii. Plasmapheresis, if blood donors are available.

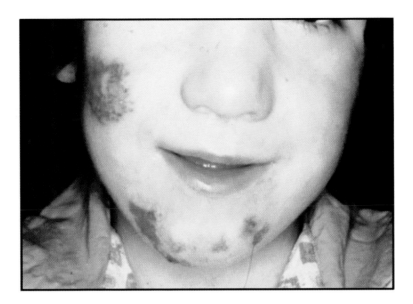

This young girl developed one lesion over her right cheek first and was pyrexial as well.

1. What abnormalities do you see?
2. What is the diagnosis?
3. What is the treatment?

ANSWERS

1. There are erythematous, irregular, raised lesions over the cheek and both side of chin.
2. Impetigo contagiosa.
3. The treatment includes:
    i. Erythromycin 250 mg thrice daily.
    ii. Cephalexin 50 mg/kg/ 24 hours in divided doses.
    iii. Cloxacillin 250 mg 6 hourly.
    iv. Recurrent impetigo is treated with rifampicin 600 mg daily or intranasal mupirocin ointment daily for 5 days.
    v. Topical mupirocin ointment (Bactroban) thrice daily for 10 days is also recommended.

    NB: Topical agents are not as good as systemic antibiotics.

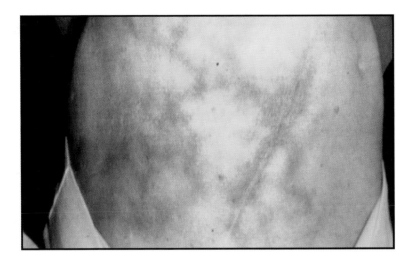

This patient had pain in abdomen.
1. What two abnormalities do you see?
2. What name is given to this abnormality?
3. How does it differ from a similar rash in autoimmune disorders?

ANSWERS

1. There is a scar mark over the right lumbar area. The skin in the same area is blotchy and is dark brown in colour with a lacy pattern.
2. Erythema ab igne. This patient had pain and used heat fomentation for relief, which caused this pigmentation. Later on he was operated leading to the scar mark.
3. It should be differentiated from livedo reticularis (see page 28).

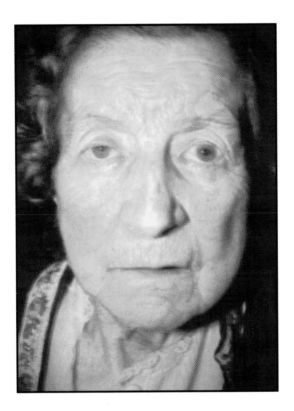

Look at this slide.
1. What abnormalities are shown in this slide?
2. What is the diagnosis?
3. Name few causes of this abnormality.

ANSWERS

1. There is partial ptosis on right with smaller palpebral fissure (enophthalmos) and constricted pupil on the right side (meiosis).
2. Right Horner's syndrome.
3. The causes include:
   a. Trauma – injury to cervical sympathetic ganglia.
   b. Post-surgical (iatrogenic).
   c. Wallenberg's syndrome- posterior inferior cerebellar artery (PICA).
   d. Syringomyelia/syringobulbia.

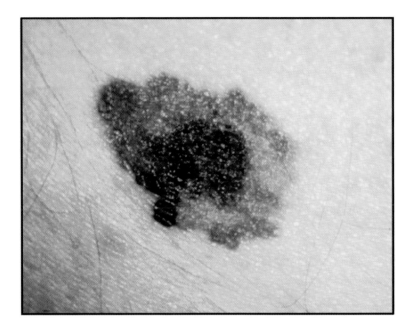

This is an itchy lesion, which bleeds sometimes.
1. What abnormality do you see?
2. What is the diagnosis?
3. What is meant by ABCDE in context with this abnormality?

ANSWERS

1. There is an area of hyperpigmention with irregular borders.
2. Malignant melanoma.
3. ABCDE is explained as follow:
   A. **A**symmetry.
   B. Irregular **B**orders.
   C. **C**olour variegation, i.e. different colours in the same lesion.
   D. **D**iameter of the lesion.
   E. **E**nlargement (rapid) of the lesion.

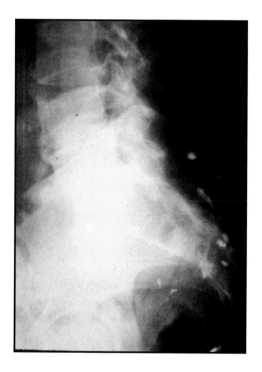

This X-ray is of a sailor who had some treatment in the past.
1. What is shown here?
2. What is the diagnosis?
3. What may be the differential diagnosis?

ANSWERS

1. This radiograph shows multiple, dense opacities of different shapes in the soft tissue of the hip.
2. Syphilis: Bismuth injections were at one time given in the gluteal area for the treatment of syphilis.
3. Cysticercosis: *Taenia solium* larvae while migrating in the muscle planes become dead and calcified giving such appearance.

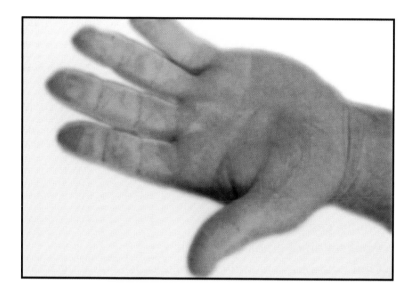

This patient felt discomfort in winter season.
1. What abnormality is shown here?
2. What is the diagnosis?
3. What is the treatment?

ANSWERS

1. There are blanched out white areas involving fingers and palm of the left hand.
2. Raynaud's phenomenon.
3. Management includes:

General Measures

    i. Avoid cold exposure.
    ii. Wear thermal gloves.
    iii. Avoid trauma.
    iv. Smoke cessation.
    v. Application of emollients on skin.
    vi. Oral beta-blockers and ergot alkaloids should be avoided.

Vasodilators

    i. Low dose nifedipine sustained release 30 mg daily orally.
    ii. Topical or oral nitroglycerine.
    iii. Serotonin reuptake inhibitors (SRI) fluoxetine 20 mg daily is also effective.
    iv. Aspirin in low dose.

Surgery

    i. Bypass for severe Raynaud's phenomenon.
    ii. Sympathectomy.

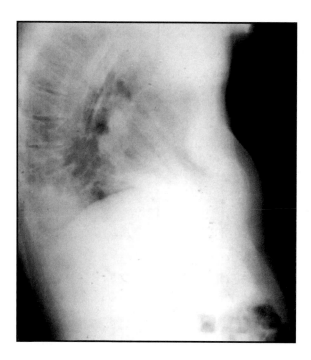

This old man had aches and pains all over and felt pain in front of his chest while breathing. He was anaemic and had raised ESR.

1. What abnormality is shown?
2. What might be the diagnosis?
3. What is the treatment?

ANSWERS

1. There is resorption of the sternum leading to sinking in front of the chest. There is marked kyphosis also.
2. Multiple myeloma.
3. Management of multiple myeloma, as a general principle includes the following:

General Measures

- Correction of dehydration.
- Correction of anaemia.
- Correction of hypercalcaemia with bisphosphonates, (e.g. editronate 7.5 mg/kg for three days) and steroids.
- Bone pain is helped by radiotherapy.
- Pathological fractures are treated by orthopaedic intervention.
- Renal involvement managed by peritoneal or haemodialysis.
- Cord compression dealt with dexamethasone and/or radio-therapy.
- Hyperviscosity syndrome is managed by plasmapheresis.

Specific Measures

- Melphalan (Alkeran) in a dose of 10 mg daily for five days with a 9 days rest. The cycle is repeated on the 14th day and this course is continued for total of 6 months.
- Corticosteroids, i.e. Prednisolone (Deltacortil) is also given as an adjuvant therapy in a dose of 40-60 mg daily for 6 months and the dose is tapered off gradually.
- Other options include cyclophosphamide, interferon-α, interferon-γ, interleukin-4 and tretinoin.

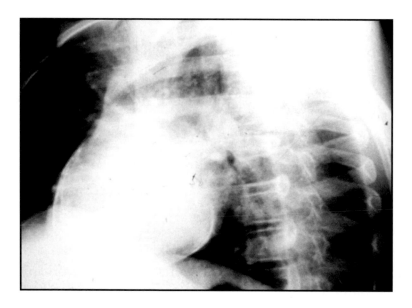

This patient had difficulty in breathing and engorged neck veins.
1. Describe the abnormality.
2. What is the diagnosis?
3. What treatment can be offered?

ANSWERS

1. This is a chest X-ray showing left lateral view of the chest demonstrating calcification of pericardium.
2. Constrictive pericarditis.
3. The initial treatment consists of gentle diuresis and then surgical removal of pericardium (pericardiotomy).

NB: In the past tuberculosis was the most common cause but now the process follows radiation therapy, cardiac surgery or viral pericarditis or histoplasmosis (less common). There is a rapid "y" descent in the JVP called Kussmaul's sign. Pulsus paradoxus is unusual. Atrial fibrillation is common association.

Other investigations include echocardiography, CT scan and MRI.

The differential diagnoses are restrictive cardiomyopathy and cardiac temponade.

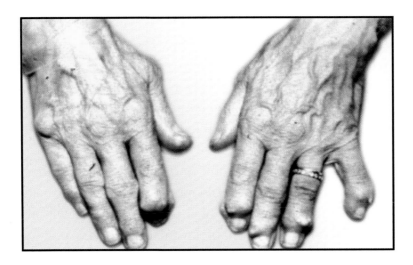

This patient passed a couple of stones in his urine.

1. Describe the abnormality in this picture.
2. What is the diagnosis?
3. How would you confirm it?
4. What treatment is advised?

ANSWERS

1. There are multiple, irregular, subcutaneous nodules at the distal interphalangeal joints with deformity. The nodules are yellowish in colour.
2. Chronic tophaceous gout.
3. Aspiration of the tophi and examination under the microscope for negatively birefringent needle like crystals found free and in the neutrophils.
4. Tophi can be made to shrink and disappear altogether with allopurinol therapy. One should maintain a serum uric acid level less than 5 mg/dl. Addition of a uricosuric agent will also be helpful. Surgical excision of large tophi offers mechanical improvement in selected deformities.

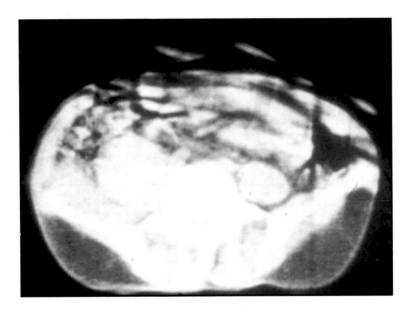

This patient had a swelling in his right groin.
1. What is this investigation?
2. What does it show?
3. What is the treatment?

ANSWERS

1. This is a slide of CT scan taken at the level of L_5 S_1, showing right sided thickened iliacus and psoas muscles.
2. Right sided ileopsoas abscess.
3. The treatment is drainage of the abscess and send for histo-pathology and microbiology. If it is tuberculous then one should start standard anti tuberculous treatment (ATT).

NB: Most of students confuse the oval opacities on both sides of vertebrae with kidneys, but the important points to note are that there is no medullary shadows of the kidneys and kidneys are not present at this level, i.e. in relation with iliacus bone which is far below the kidney level (kidneys are present at L1-L2 level).

SLIDE - 98

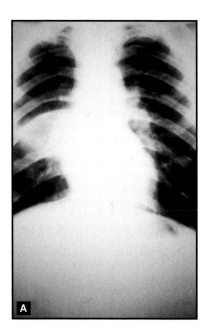 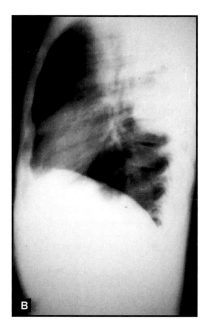

This patient had deafness and hypertension. Look at these X-rays.
1. What is shown in A?
2. What is shown in B?
3. What may be the diagnosis?

ANSWERS

1. There is a homogenous triangular opacity in the right middle zone which seems attached to right border of heart (Silhouette's sign).
2. This is the lateral view showing a normal cardiac shadow but a rounded homogenous opacity is seen over the vertebral column.
3. A para-vertebral tumour. In this case the patient had a neurofibroma and the underlying diagnosis was von Recklinghausen's disease.

NB: Such X-ray especially (A) can be misinterpreted as right middle lobe pneumonia as there is a Silhouette's sign but it is important to get a lateral view to actually confirm it or rule out other causes.

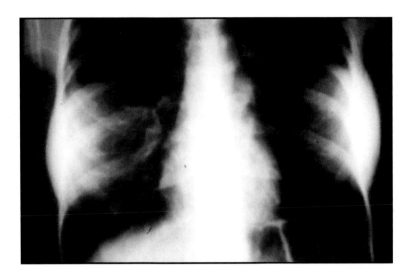

This patient was a symptomatic.
1. Describe the abnormality.
2. What is the diagnosis?
3. What complications can occur?

ANSWERS

1. There are bilateral symmetrical opacities in the middle zones of both lung fields and they are also bulging out from the chest wall.
2. Silicon breast implants.
3. Complications include the following:

Immediate Complications

- Haematoma.
- Acute or subacute infections.
- Hypoaesthesia in and around nipple.

Delayed Complications

- Capsule formation.
- Deshaping of breast due to fibrosis in the capsule.

NB: At times it was thought that the incidence of lymphoma and auto-immune disorders were more common but a few long-term studies have failed to confirm that.

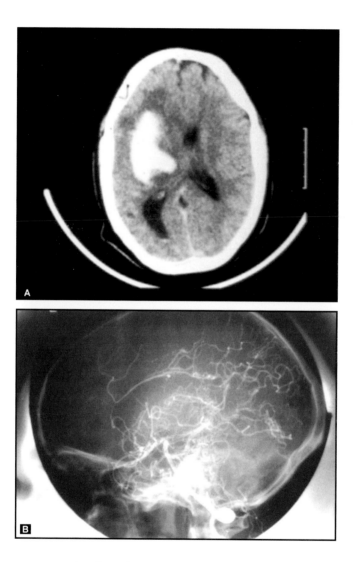

This young man had sudden onset of headache and developed right-sided weakness.

1. What is this investigation and what is shown in picture A?
2. What is this investigation and what is shown in picture B?
3. What is the diagnosis?
4. What is the treatment?

ANSWERS

1. CT scan brain shows a hyper dense area in the left parietal lobe with mid line shift to the opposite side.
2. Vertebral artery angiogram showing posterior circulation only.
3. Moya moya disease.
4. Management primarily is symptomatic and supportive. Evacuation of haematoma is advised if there is rapid deterioration in neurological signs.

   As regards moya moya disease itself, procedures like perivascular sympathectomy of the cervical part of carotid artery, superior cervical ganglion sympathectomy, arterial anastomosis and intracranial transplantation of omentum have been tried but their effectiveness is not proven.

   Prognosis is variable and depends on the severity of the clinical picture.

   NB: Moya moya disease should be suspected as a potential cause of cerebral ischaemia or intracerebral haemorrhage in young adults although it is a very rare entity in South East Asians and Caucasians.

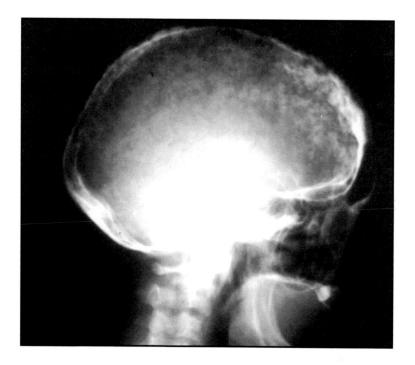

This patient had fractured her right femur and had renal lithiasis.
1. What is shown in this slide?
2. What is the diagnosis?
3. What other complications may occur?
4. What is the treatment?

ANSWERS

1. There are diffuse areas of lesser bone density with areas of normal bone density. This is called pepper pot appearance.
2. Hyperparathyroidism.
3. Acute pancreatitis, peptic ulceration, corneal calcification, depression, hypersomnia, pruritis, psychosis and even coma.
4. Surgical excision of parathyroid adenoma if present. Later on calcium and vitamin D supplementation is necessary.

Other measures include treatment of hypercalcaemia with high fluid intake. Bisphosphonates are used as well.

Avoid vitamin D, calcium and thiazide diuretics.

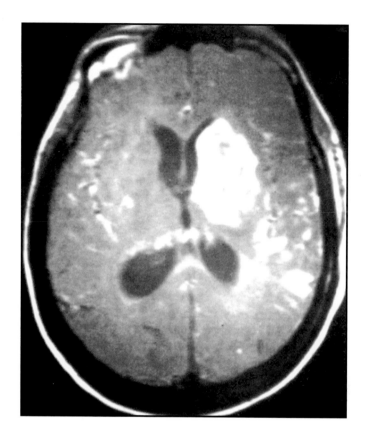

This patient had headaches, low-grade fever and vomiting.
1. What is this investigation?
2. What does it show?
3. What is the diagnosis?
4. What is the treatment?

ANSWERS

1. This is CT scan of brain.
2. It shows an irregular hyper dense area in the right parietal lobe with compression of the anterior horn of the right ventricle. There are scattered hyper dense areas in between the sulci.
3. Tuberculoma secondary to tuberculous meningitis.
4. Anti tubercular therapy but if tuberculoma is causing pressure symptoms then it should be removed surgically.

SLIDE - 103

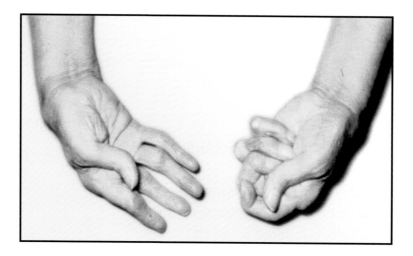

This patient complained of early morning stiffness.
1. What abnormalities do you see?
2. What is the diagnosis?
3. Name few eye complications.

ANSWERS

1. There is swan neck deformity of the fingers of the right hand with Z- deformity of the right thumb. There is flexion deformity of the digits of left hand with Z-deformity of the left thumb.
2. Rheumatoid arthritis.
3. The eye complications are:
   a. Due to disease itself:
      - Episcleritis, keratoconjunctivitis sicca.
      - Scleritis.
      - Scleromalacia perforans.
   b. Due to therapy for rheumatoid arthritis:
      - Steroids induced cataracts.
      - Chloroquine salt cause retinal toxicity.

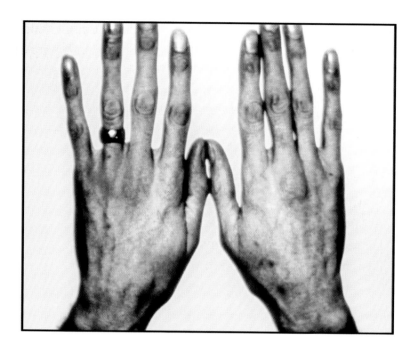

This man complained of breathlessness and had a precordial murmur.

1. What is the abnormality?
2. What name is given to it?
3. What is the diagnosis?
4. What other clinical signs are associated with this diagnosis?

ANSWERS

1. These fingers are cyanosed and longer than normal.
2. Arachanodactyly.
3. Marfan's syndrome.
4. The other associated clinical signs are:
    i. High arched palate.
    ii. Tall stature.
    iii. Long arm span.
    iv. Laxity of joints – Steinberg's sign.
    v. Spontaneous pneumothorax.
    vi. Aortic valve incompetence.
    vii. Dissecting aortic aneurysms.
    viii. Dislocation or sub-luxation of lens.

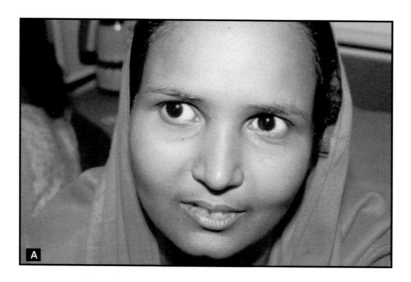

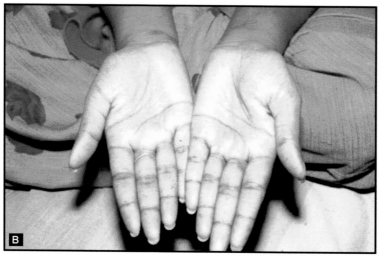

These two slides are from the same patients who complained of tiredness and giddy spells.

    1. What is shown in slide A?

ANSWERS

1. The face of a young girl with dark complexion especially over the temples and around mouth
2. The palmar creases are dark against pale palms.
3. Addison's disease – as she has giddy spells and extreme tiredness (two of the commonest features).
4. The bed side examination will include:
   a. Postural hypotension.
   b. Buccal pigmentation.

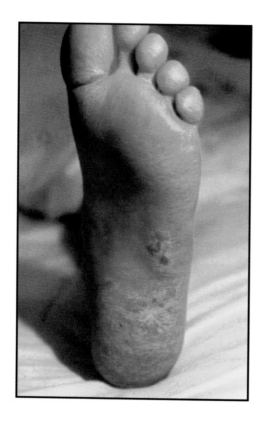

This young man had urethral discharge and conjunctivitis.
1. What is shown here?
2. What is the diagnosis?
3. What is the treatment?

212 Slide Interpretation in Clinical Medicine

ANSWERS

1. There are multiple hyperkeratotic lesions over the left sole more marked in the heel area. This is called keratoderma blenorrhagica.
2. Reiter's syndrome.
3. The mainstay of treatment is:
    i. Non-steroidal anti-inflammatory agents.
    ii. Tetracycline 250 mg q.d.s for 3 months to these patients if associated with *C. trachomatis* infection.
    iii. Anti-TNF-α agents (Etanercept and infliximab) are reasonable therapies for patients with refractory disease.

NB: Reiter's syndrome is characterized by oligoarthritis (less than three joints involved), conjunctivitis, urethritis, circinate balanitis, and keratoderma blenorrhagica and mouth ulcers. It usually follows dysentery or sexually transmitted diseases. It is associated with HLA-B 27 in 80% of white patients and 50-60% blacks.

The causative organism is *Chlamydia trachomatis* or perhaps *Ureaplasma urealyticum*. M: F ratio is 1:1 after enteric infection but 9:1 after sexually transmitted infection. Fever, weight loss, muco-cutaneous lesions may include balanitis, stomatitis and keratoderma blenorrhagica which is to be differentiated from psoriasis.

Carditis and aortic regurgitation may occur. Sacroiliac joint is commonly involved. This is differentiated from gonococcal arthritis, rheumatoid arthritis, ankylosing spondylitis and psoriatic arthritis. Association with HIV has been debated.

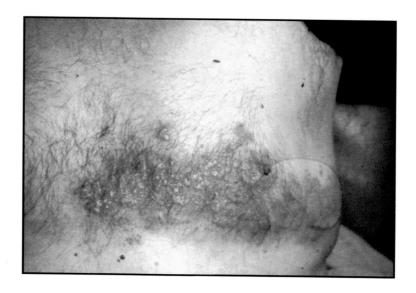

The patient developed a very painful rash over his trunk.

    1. Describe this rash.

    2. What is it?

    3. What is the treatment?

    4. What complications may occur?

ANSWERS

1. There is vesiculo-papular rash on the front of chest over left side and is not crossing the mid line.
2. Herpes zoster of the thoracic area.
3. The treatment includes:
    i. Systemic acyclovir.
    ii. Topical acyclovir.
    iii. Systemic antibiotics.
    iv. Calamine lotion topically.
4. Super added infections.
    Post herpetic neuralgia.

SLIDE - 108

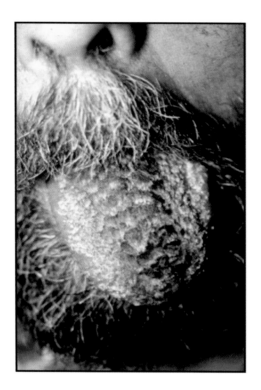

This patient was unkempt.
1. Describe the abnormality.
2. What name is given to this abnormality?
3. What is the cause?
4. What is the treatment?

ANSWERS

1. There is blackening of the tongue with coating over the surface.
2. Black hairy tongue – it is due to black discolouration of the papillae over the tongue which stands out prominently like hairs.
3. Candida nigra – it is a fungal infection especially in patients who are unkempt and do not take care of their oral hygiene.
4. Antifungal agents, i.e. nystatin or fluconazole.

SLIDE - 109

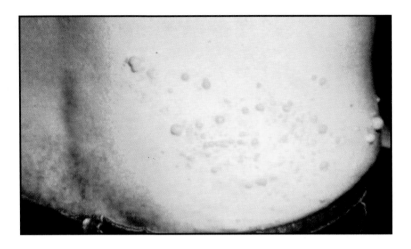

This patient was symptomatic but had few freckles in both axillae.

1. Describe the abnormality.
2. What is it?
3. Name few complications of the primary diagnosis.

ANSWERS

1. There are nodular swellings of variable sizes distributed on one side of the right flank. Few are sessile and few are pedunculated.
2. Segmental neurofibromatosis.
3. The clinical feature include:
   i. Café au lait spots.
   ii. Lisch's nodules.
   iii. Meningiomas.
   iv. Acoustic neuroma.
   v. Glioma.
   vi. Kyphoscoliosis.
   vii. Pheochromocytoma.

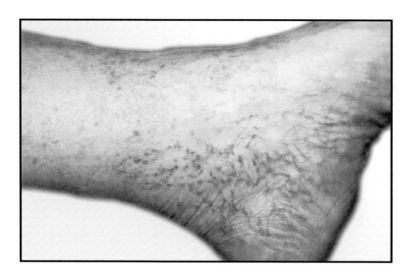

This patient is asymptomatic.

1. What is the abnormality? Describe it.
2. What name is given to it?
3. What is the treatment?

ANSWERS

1. There are fine blood vessels visible over the medial aspect of left ankle. These are in the from of a network and are blanchable.
2. This is called ankle flare.
3. There is no treatment as it is a normal finding in some normal subjects.

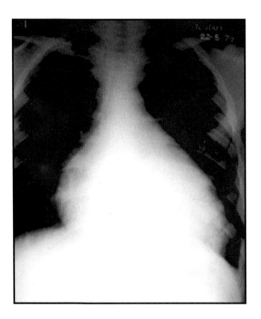

This patient was breathless even at rest.

1. Describe the abnormality on this X-ray.
2. What is the diagnosis?
3. What is the treatment?
4. What can cause this appearance?

ANSWERS

1. The cardiac size is enlarged with smooth cardiac borders, leading to a pear shaped heart.
2. Pericardial effusion.
3. The treatment is pericardiocentesis, under echocardiographic control.
4. Causes of pericardial effusion include:
     i. Any infective pericarditis.
    ii. Uraemia.
   iii. Postmyocardial infarction.
    iv. Rheumatoid arthritis.
     v. Hypothyroidism.
    vi. Malignancy.
   vii. Trauma.
  viii. Post-cardiotomy syndrome.
    ix. Dressler's syndrome.

SLIDE - 112

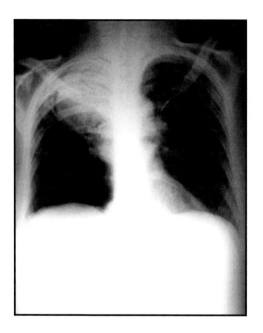

This patient had haemoptysis.
1. What is shown in the X-ray? What is the diagnosis?
2. How would you confirm it radiologically?
3. Name three complications.
4. What is the treatment?

ANSWERS

1. There is rounded homogenous opacity in the right upper zone with a crescent of air around it. It is an apergilloma or fungus ball (mycetoma).
2. The confirmation is by taking the X-ray with a change in position, i.e. right lateral or left lateral decubitus view. The ball is free to move in the cavity and crescent of air changes its location. Other option is to go for a tomogram to see the ball clearly.
3. Haemoptysis.
   Fungaemia.
   Bronchial hyperactivity.
4. The treatment includes use of antifungal agents including itraconazole in a dose of 200 mg daily for 3 months. Amphotericin B can be used intralesionally as well. The definitive treatment is surgical resection.

SLIDE - 113

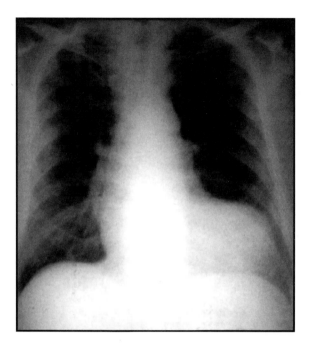

This patient had orthopnoea.

1. What is shown in this picture?
2. Why is this patient short of breath?
3. What ECG changes you might expect?

ANSWERS

1. The cardiac shadow is enlarged and the tip of left ventricle is almost reaching the left chest wall. This is due to left ventricular aneurysm.
2. The aneurysmal dilatation leads to a dyskinetic ventricular segment, resulting in increased pre-load thus causing congestion in the lungs and breathlessness.
3. The ECG usually shows Q-waves with persistent elevation of ST-segment with convexity upwards.

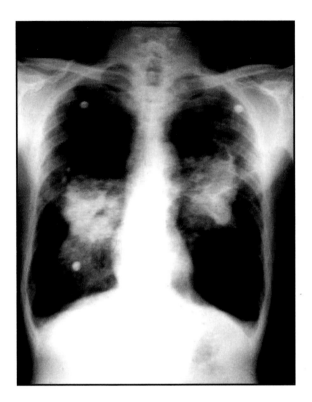

This X-ray is from a coal miner.

1. Describe the abnormalities.
2. What is the diagnosis?
3. What other complications may develop?

ANSWERS

1. There are bilateral non-homogeneous opacities in both hilar areas. The rest of the lungs are hyperlucent. Both the diaphragmatic domes are depressed and are at the same level. Electrodes for monitoring are also visible.
2. Progressive massive fibrosis (PMF).
3. The complications include:
   • Respiratory failure.
   • Recurrent chest infections.

SLIDE - 115

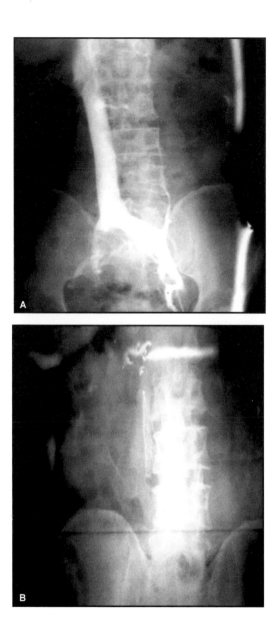

This patient had tender, swollen and warm right leg.
1. What is shown in A?
2. What procedure has taken place in B?
3. What are the complications of this procedure?

ANSWERS

1. This is an inferior vena caval venogram showing occlusion of the right common iliac vein. The left common iliac vein is filling properly.
2. A vena caval filter called Kimray-Greenfield filter is lodged in the inferior vena cava.
3. The complications include:
   - Inability of filter to open completely.
   - Filter does not lodge properly at all.
   - Lodges in the wrong place.
   - Floats through to the right ventricle.
   - Aorto-caval communication (window).
   - Erosion of the filter.
   - Migration of the filter after dislodging.
   - Inferior vena caval obstruction.
   - Venous thrombosis at the site of filter insertion

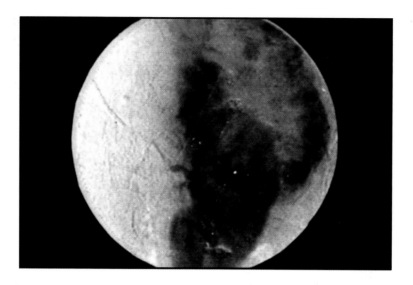

This patient was hypertensive.

1. What is this investigation?
2. What does it show?
3. What is the diagnosis?
4. What is the treatment?

ANSWERS

1. This is a left renal arteriogram.
2. It outlines the kidney well along with a diffuse contrast shadow over the upper pole of the kidney.
3. Left adrenal mass (tumour).
4. Surgical resection of the tumour with replacement therapy of the hormones.

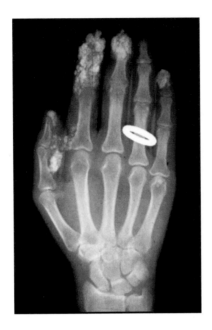

This patient had dysphagia.

1. Describe this X-ray.
2. What is the diagnosis?
3. What other complications you know of this disease?

ANSWERS

1. There are hyper dense, irregular opacities in the subcutaneous tissue of the right thumb and index, middle and little finger.
2. Calcinosis cutis.
3. It is associated with auto-immune or mixed connective tissue diseases, e.g. systemic sclerosis or CREST which includes
   - Calcinosis cutis.
   - Raynaud's phenomenon.
   - Oesophageal dysmotility.
   - Sclerodactyly.
   - Telangiectasia.

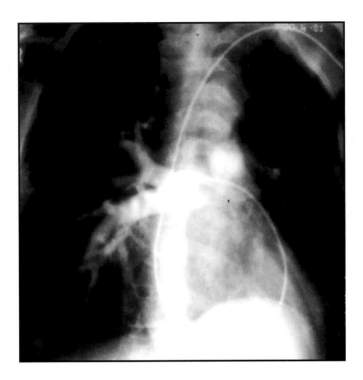

This patient collapsed on the ward after he was admitted for exploratory laparotomy.

1. What is this investigation?
2. What does it show?
3. What is the diagnosis?
4. What treatment would you plan?

ANSWERS

1. This is a pulmonary angiogram.
2. It shows that there is no flow of the contrast towards left main pulmonary artery.
3. Massive pulmonary embolism
4. The treatment includes:
   - Supportive care including oxygen therapy and inotropic support.
   - Thrombolytic therapy including intravenous heparin, streptokinase or recombinant tissue plasminogen activator (TPA).
   - Pulmonary embolectomy as specific therapy.
   - Preventive therapy includes long-term anti-coagulation and inferior vena caval filters.

SLIDE - 119

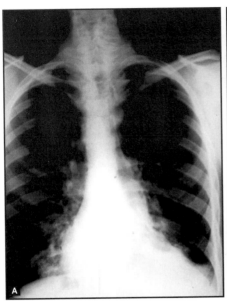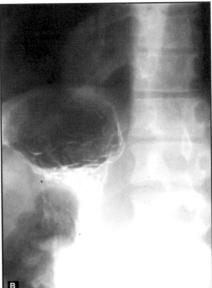

This patient had recurrent attacks of sinusitis and was infertile.
1. What is shown in A?
2. What is shown in B?
3. What is the diagnosis?
4. Where is the basic pathology?
5. What is the treatment?

ANSWERS

1. There is dextrocardia and the air bubble of the stomach is under the right dome of the diaphragm.
2. It is a barium meal showing that the stomach is on the right side.
3. Kartagener's syndrome—there is situs inversus, i.e. total transposition of vessels as well.
4. There is defect in the rotation of the foregut.
5. There is no curative treatment. It is basically symptomatic.

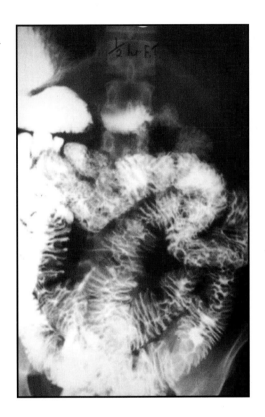

This patient had watery diarrhoea.
   1. What is this investigation?
   2. What does it show?
   3. What is the diagnosis?

ANSWERS

1. This is a barium follow through examination.
2. It shows that mucosal pattern of the small bowel is feathery and there is oedema of the mucosal folds.
3. Lymphangiectasia of the small bowel.

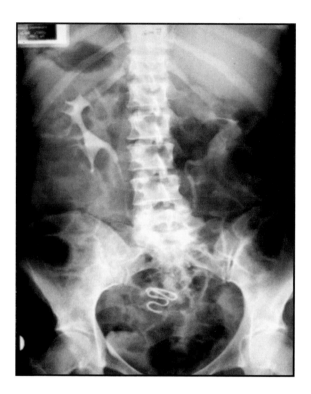

This patient was hypertensive and had renal failure.
1. Can you guess the sex of this patient?
2. What abnormalities do you see in this slide?
3. What is the diagnosis?
4. What treatment is offered?

ANSWERS

1. This is a female patient.
2. This is an intravenous urogram showing bilaterally distorted pelvicalyceal system of both kidneys along with a lippes loop in the bony pelvis.
3. Polycystic kidney disease.
4. Management includes:
    - Control of blood pressure.
    - Renal replacement therapy.
    - Renal transplantation.

SLIDE - 122

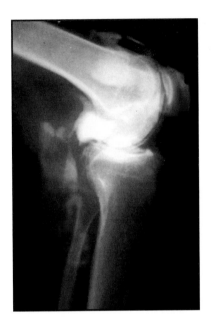

This patient had swollen right leg after walking routinely.
1. What is this investigation?
2. What does it show?
3. What is the diagnosis?
4. What is the treatment?

ANSWERS

1. This is an arthrogram.
2. It shows that the dye is spilling over in the popliteal area way down towards the upper part of the lower leg.
3. It is a ruptured Baker's cyst.
4. Treatment is mostly symptomatic.

SLIDE - 123

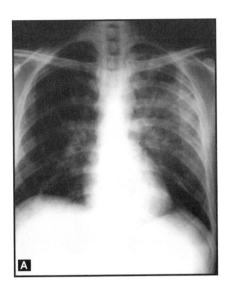 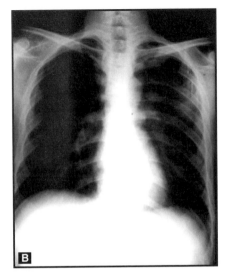

These two X-rays belong to a drug addict patient who presented
with fever, cough and severe prostration and had some treatment.

1. What is shown in A?
2. What is shown in B?
3. What is the diagnosis?
4. What treatment is recommended?

ANSWERS

1. There is bilateral infiltration in the middle zones of the lungs more marked on the left side.
2. This X-ray chest appears almost normal.
3. Pneumocystis carinii pneumonia (PCP).
4. High dose cotrimoxazole (sulphamethoxazole + trimethoprim) for 14 days. Intravenous pentamadine for 21 days is also beneficial. Addition of systemic steroids may improve the outcome.

SLIDE - 124

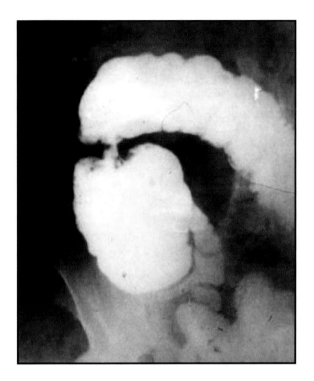

This patient had history of weight loss and passed blood per rectum on three occasions.
1. What is this investigation?
2. Describe the abnormality and what name is given to this appearance?
3. What is the management?

ANSWERS

1. This is a barium enema.
2. There is a filling defect in the ascending colon which is like a stricture and there is marked "shouldering". This is called apple core appearance. It is usually due to carcinoma of colon.
3. Management includes:
   - Resection of the primary colonic cancer is the treatment of choice if this is possible. Even patients with metastatic disease can benefit from resection as it improves quality of life by reducing the likelihood of bleeding and intestinal obstruction.
   - Adjuvant chemotherapy with fluorouracil along with or without leucovorin has been used widely for palliation without improving survival. Combination therapy with fluorouracil, leucovorin and irinotecan provides significant improvement in tumour response rate (40%) and overall survival of 15 months as compared with fluorouracil and leucovorin alone.
   - Patients, whose disease progresses despite therapy, meticulous efforts at palliative care are essential.

NB: Patients, who have undergone surgery, should be closely monitored for recurrence. Yearly colonoscopy, CT scanning and chest radiography was recommended at one time but currently patients should be evaluated every 3-6 months for 3-5 years with history and detailed physical examination, faecal occult blood, liver function tests and CEA estimation.

Colonoscopy should be performed within 6-12 months of operation for recurrence and then every 3-5 years to look for metachronous tumours.

It should be understood that the stage of the disease at the time of presentation is most important. The survival for stage I is >90%; stage II, > 70%; stage III, 33-67%; and stage IV has a survival less than 50%.

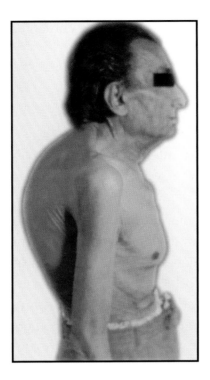

This patient complained of shortness of breath and was coughing up purulent sputum.

1. Describe the abnormality on this slide.
2. What complications can occur?
3. How do you differentiate it from gibbus deformity?

ANSWERS

1. The back of the chest is uniformly curved backwards and this is called kyphosis.
2. The complications include:
   - Back ache.
   - Exertional dyspnoea.
   - Basal atelectasis.
   - Recurrent chest infections.
   - Restrictive lung disease.
   - Cor pulmonale.
   - Early osteopenia, osteoporosis and vertebral collapse.
3. In "gibbus" deformity, there is an acute angulation of the thoracic spine at its mid level and it is due to an infective process, i.e. caries spine or osteomyelitis or trauma resulting in vertebral fracture. However, in kyphosis there is a uniform curvature of the dorsal spine and there is no acute angulation.

INDEX